Dying

Considerations Concerning the Passage from Life to Death

Lawrence Whytehead
Paul Chidwick
editors

Task Force on Human Life
Anglican Church of Canada

The Anglican Book Centre
Toronto, Canada

Published by
The Anglican Book Centre
600 Jarvis Street
Toronto, Ontario
Canada M4Y 2J6

Printed in Canada
ISBN 0-919030-53-X

Contents

Foreword

As factual knowledge and technological skills continue to expand in our world, issues relating to life and death become increasingly complex. This is particularly true in the realm of moral decision making. When are we prolonging life, and when are we prolonging dying? These are difficult questions, and behind them lie even more dificult ones — how do we define life, and how do we define death?

What is the role of the church in these complex matters which are so close to each of us? How does this report relate to that role?

I believe the role of the church is to encourage people to strive to know and to do the will of God in the situations they are called upon to face. In this role the Anglican communion affirms that there are three vital factors in determining the will of God — scripture, the tradition of the church, and conscience enlightened by reason. The individual in the community of the church must be prepared to struggle with the difficult decisions which arise, assisted by the thinking of the community, under the leading of the Holy Spirit.

This report is *not* a definitive statement setting forth official church positions. Rather it is a document designed to help persons within the Christian community, (which is set within a wider social order), to make more responsible choices and decisions under God as he has revealed himself to us in Jesus Christ. It is not to be seen as the last word, but as a contribution to individuals and the church, as together we seek to be faithful to our calling "to follow our Saviour Christ and to be made like unto him."

May it provide help and support as people struggle to be faithful; may it lead to further thought and consideration as more knowledge becomes available.

Edward W. Scott
Primate

Preface and Acknowledgements

The Twenty-Seventh General Synod of the Anglican Church of Canada, meeting in Quebec City, 12–19 June 1975, requested the Primate to reappoint the Task Force on Human Life "to prepare a report on death and dying, including the extension of life by mechanical and other means." Subsequently it was decided that a number of independent study groups should be set up across Canada and that their discussions on this subject should be reported to the Rev Canon Paul Chidwick, who would act as a liaison between these committees.

An interim report was presented to the Twenty-Eighth General Synod of the Anglican Church of Canada, meeting in Calgary in August 1977. The report was prepared by a study group in Winnipeg and compiled under the joint editorship of Dr Lawrence Whytehead and the Rev Canon Paul Chidwick. The members of the group were as follows:

Dr Lawrence Whytehead, Surgeon (Chairman)
Health Sciences Centre
Winnipeg, Manitoba

The Rev Canon Paul F. Chidwick, Parish Priest
St Mary's Walkerville
Windsor, Ontario

Dr Robert Blanchard, Surgeon
Health Sciences Centre
Winnipeg, Manitoba

Arthur Braid, Lawyer, Professor
Faculty of Law, University of Manitoba
Winnipeg, Manitoba

Muriel Burry, Head Nurse
Neurosurgical Ward, Health Sciences Centre
Winnipeg, Manitoba

The Rev David Clark, Chaplain
Health Sciences Centre
Winnipeg, Manitoba

The Rev Ronald J. Con (deceased)
Presbyterian Minister & Social Development Officer
Winnipeg, Manitoba

The Rev Robert English, Parish Priest
Church of the Good Shepherd,
Winnipeg, Manitoba

Dr Leonard La Rue, General Practitioner
Manitoba

Dr David Skelton, former Director
Department of Geriatric Medicine,
St Boniface Hospital
Winnipeg, Manitoba

Penelope Washbourn, Professor
Department of Religion
St John's College, University of Manitoba
Winnipeg, Manitoba

The General Synod, after discussion, sent the interim report back to the study group for rewriting (Resolution 87). The membership of the group was augmented by:

The Right Reverend Barry Valentine, Bishop of Rupert's Land

Before the task of rewriting was begun, the Study Group consulted with the following theologians:

The Rev T. Appleton,
Faculty of Divinity
St John's College
Assistant in the parish of All Saints
Winnipeg, Manitoba

The Rev J. M. Badertscher,
Department of Religious Studies,
University of Winnipeg
Winnipeg, Manitoba

The Rev Canon J. R. Brown, Warden
St John's College
Winnipeg, Manitoba

The Rev G. W. Ladd, Parish Priest
Hodgson-Peguis Group, Diocese of Rupert's Land

The Rev J. C. Ridd,
Department of Religious Studies,
University of Winnipeg
Winnipeg, Manitoba

The study group extends sincere thanks to these consultants for their invaluable help.

The Anglican Consultative Council at its third meeting in March 1976, when considering "the sanctity of human life," emphasized that the Church has a heavy responsibility to offer guidance to its members and to the society in which it seeks to witness to the truth. Pointing out that "moral theology recognizes an unqualified imperative: to love one's neighbour as oneself," it insisted that "each individual has the responsibility of working out the application of this principle to the particular circumstances in question." It suggested that answerability and responsibility to God and to their fellow men is one characteristic distinguishing persons from other created beings and firmly stated that "the Church must give every possible support to those who have to make these difficult decisions."[1]

In the spirit of these statements and within the terms of reference of the Task Force on Human Life, the revised report discusses relevant personal, social, medical, and legal issues, with emphasis on underlying theological insights. It is offered to the general body of the Church and, indeed, to all members of society, trusting that it will help them to appreciate the problems and dilemmas involved in the care of those who are "sick unto death." In particular, we believe that doctors, nurses, and others of the medical team, as well as the clergy, will find in these pages support, understanding, and guidance for the care of dying persons and their families. While our words are not directed to theologians, we hope that they will be in agreement with what we have written. To all we would say that we have tried to present a full picture of the problems posed by death in our technological age. We have attempted not to give answers, though the reader may detect bias, but to assist each individual to work out his or her own position on the problems involved.

It should be made clear that the report as a whole is accepted by all members of the study group as a reasonable statement of all aspects that must be taken into account in this subject. This is not to say, however, that each member endorses every detail of the report, or the implications which may be deduced from some passages.

In addition to the theological consultants, the study group wishes to acknowledge communications from countless individuals and groups across Canada, and even from south of the 49th parallel. They expressed views ranging across the entire spectrum of thought and opinion on our present subject. Some openly condemned the interim report, others endorsed it, but the majority expressed deep interest and offered comments, above all praising the attempt to bring the problems of dying today before the Church and society. There were too many communications to be answered individually by the editors, but to all who took the trouble to write or speak, privately or publicly, the study group offers a sincere "thank you." Clearly, with such a variety of opinions and suggestions, only a few were incorporated in the revised report, but whether or not the individual reader can detect the influence of his or her point of view, the response to the interim report had a profound effect on the study group and the editors.

We wish to express our gratitude to Phyllis Creighton for reviewing the manuscript, for her many suggestions for developing some aspects and for making it more readable. Dr Cope Schwenger also reviewed the material and made useful recommendations to improve the presentation. Douglas Hodgkinson has prepared a study guide for groups wishing to examine and discuss important issues raised in the report. As well, a number of secretaries were involved in typing the drafts and numerous revisions, and thus assisted in the production of the written report. To each of them also, we extend our thanks.

1
The Problem and Man's Response

Dying Today

The remark that people are more afraid of dying than of death itself has become commonplace. The request many people make today is to be allowed to die with dignity. Unfortunately there are many factors which make it difficult for them to attain what they want. Dr Balfour Mount outlines some of the problems.

> Approximately 70% of Canadians now die in institutions. There is increasing evidence that these patients and their families experience a wide variety of critical problems that usually go unrecognized by those responsible for their care. The terminally ill patient, instead of receiving sympathetic understanding and expertise in meeting his medical and emotional needs, may encounter isolation and depersonalization.... As death approaches, interaction between patient and staff becomes strained and patient care is affected.... Physicians visit with decreasing frequency the longer a patient is hospitalized, and nursing care decreases as a patient's death becomes imminent. It takes longer for a nurse to answer the bell rung by a dying patient than by a patient expected to recover. Isolation, suspicion and distrust develop owing to the lack of communication between patients, family members, nurses and physicians. This is fostered by physicians' reluctance to inform the patient of the diagnosis and prognosis, a natural preference to treat disease rather than to deal with personal and social problems, and an endemic denial of death.[1]

Similar sentiments were expressed by the former Archbishop of Canterbury, Dr Coggan, in the 1976 Edwin Stevens Lecture of the Royal Society of Medicine. Using the words of a Roman Catholic authority, Dr Coggan indicated his own distress "at the conspiracy of silence which so often surrounds death, a silence which isolates the person who is dying and who, just because of his condition, needs the consolation of understanding companionship." He went on to assert that "this kind of thing results in putting the dying person in emotional isolation, or in treating him as though he were a child unable to take responsibility on an adult level. He thus finds himself in loose touch with people who do not communicate with him naturally and who, because of their lack of ease in the presence of impending death, fail to fulfil their share of total responsibility."[2]

There are numerous examples to illustrate the dilemma of the dying patient. One such case, described by Hugh Trowell in his book *The Unfinished Debate on Euthanasia,* is that of a doctor who had retired after a coronary thrombosis and developed cancer of the stomach.

> An operation was performed to deal with the cancer but it had spread far and wide. Part of the stomach was removed and the diagnosis was confirmed. Analgesic drugs to deaden pain and even morphine injections at night only partially controlled the pain, as the growths had spread to the spine and were pressing on the nerves. Ten days after the operation a clot of blood suddenly blocked one of the arteries of the lungs. This might have proved rapidly fatal had not an emergency operation removed the clot. The patient expressed his appreciation of the good intentions and skills of the young surgeon but asked that if other complications occurred no steps should be taken to prolong his life. He wrote a note to this effect on his case records. Two weeks later he had another coronary thrombosis but was resuscitated by the hospital's emergency team. That night his heart stopped four times; each time it was re-started artificially. He lingered on for three more weeks, but, perhaps fortunately for him, his brain was not functioning and he was unconscious. Intravenous fluids however fed him and antibiotics prevented infections. On the last day plans were made to help his failing breathing by an artificial respirator but the heart stopped before this endeavour could be realized.[3]

This is obviously an extreme example of prolonging the dying process; nevertheless, it does illustrate the problems facing both patient and doctor. The patient has no wish to live a depersonalizing existence and sees few options open to him, while the medical staff have to decide such issues as the hopelessness of the case, the real nature and meaning of the patient's wishes, and the beneficial effects of particular treatments.

There are far too many questions being asked by dying patients, next-of-kin, and doctors, that demand serious response but remain unanswered. The dying person may look for meaning in his suffering and, finding none, wishes his life would soon end. At the same time he wonders if he has any right to ask other people to hasten his death. He becomes very conscious that people are avoiding him. "The nurses don't look me in the eye, and they avoid my questions. My family used to kiss me when they left, but now they just pat my hand or wave good-bye at the door." The mature patient recognizes day by day that he is being denied those things that have always been the indicators of adulthood. No one asks him for his opinion about his health. His freedom to decide what he will do, what he will wear, where he will go, is denied. When a problem is raised about some issue in the family, he is told not to worry. There is constant denial of his role as a free, responsible individual, and as a result he may question to what extent he is still a person.

The next-of-kin may feel that the patient's suffering is unnecessarily prolonged and secretly hope that it may soon be over. They find it more and more difficult to talk with him and eventually revert to banalities about the weather and school reports. They make jokes about his relationship with the nurses and encourage him to be a "good boy" and eat up his dinner. In their minds the patient slowly becomes a child-like figure who needs to be cared for and is utterly dependent on them. In the course of time the next-of-kin may begin to regard the patient as a burden and then feel guilty about this reaction. They may question what they are doing in the room and doubt the value of their visits. Their sense of helplessness can lead to intense frustration and anger.

In cases that involve the care of a defective newborn, decision-making can be agonizing for both parents and doctors. A letter written by Robert and Peggy Stinson to the hospital authorities about the care of their baby in the Intensive Care Unit illustrates the problems. Andrew was born 15-1/2 weeks prematurely, weighed only 1 lb. 12 oz. and was in a state of painful deterioration from the start. In the course of treatment his condition worsened.

> The sad list of Andrew's afflictions, almost all of which were iatrogenic, reveals how disastrous this hospitalization was. Andrew had a months-long, unresolved case of bronchopulmonary dysplasia, sometimes referred to as "respirator lung syndrome." He was "saved" by the respirator to endure countless episodes of bradycardia and cyanosis, countless suctionings

> and tube insertions and blood samplings and blood transfusions, "saved" to develop retrolental fibroplasia, numerous infections, demineralized and fractured bones, an iatrogenic cleft palate, and, finally, as his lungs became irreparably diseased, pulmonary artery hypertension and seizures of the brain. He was, in effect, "saved" by the respirator to die five long, painful, and expensive months later of the respirator's side effects....
>
> Complicating Andrew's respiratory and nutritional difficulties was the fact that the ICU could not protect him from recurring rounds of infection. During his stay at Pediatric Hospital, Andrew suffered through a prolonged case of E. coli septicemia, related abscesses at the arterial line sites which necessitated surgical removal of gangrene and necrotic muscle down to the bone of his right leg (it was noted in the record in May that "right foot remains limited due to severed and removed muscle tissue"), several urinary tract infections, and "multiple courses of pneumonia."[4]

Andrew's parents could see no point in such sophisticated and extraordinary care, but because this care was available, the doctors had felt obliged to respond in every way possible. Both had been faced with the dilemma of deciding what was good for the child.

Further distressing difficulties arise in the care of patients in irreversible coma. Medical journals abound with cases such as the following.

> A 51-year-old man was brought to the hospital following a massive, crushing injury to the upper body, with multiple rib fractures, extensive lung contusion, hemothorax, brachial plexus avulsion, and acute venous congestion of the head and neck. The patient was responsive initially and stabilized with therapy. Continuous respirator support through a tracheostomy became necessary subsequently. On the eighth day, the patient no longer responded, had fixed, dilated pupils, and exhibited no motor activity, no reflexes, and no spontaneous respiration. Electroencephalography with maximum gain, on two occasions 48 hours apart, showed totally isoelectric tracings. Cardiovascular function and renal function continued, and the pulmonary pathology cleared. The patient was maintained in this state with parenteral fluids and continuous respirator support until sudden cardiovascular collapse occurred and death

was pronounced on the 20th hospital day. Autopsy revealed extensive degeneration of cerebral substance, inconsistent with recovery.[5]

In cases like those just described, the physicians appear to have focused their attention solely on the physical condition of the patient rather than to have taken a holistic approach encompassing the needs of the total person. Consequently many doctors are concerned that in such instances they are merely preserving biological life. Modern medical technology has forced us to consider the distinction between personal existence and biological existence. When the characteristics of personal life appear to be absent or are drifting away, the decision to withhold or withdraw treatment becomes an alternative.

In all the examples cited above there should be an over-riding concern: What sort of care will serve the good of the patient? How can we enhance his well-being as a person? These problems will never be resolved until we achieve a better understanding of what it means to be a human person. What is unique to us as persons? How can we respect this uniqueness, reverence it, and nurture it by our care? It is both appropriate and essential in a report of this kind to consider the unique characteristics that distinguish personal human life from other forms of created life. Clarification of our thinking and beliefs may provide guidance when decisions are needed concerning those who are sick or in the process of dying, decisions that must be reached by health care professionals, by the close family, and by the individual who is the centre of concern. Those who take part in such decisions will need the loving acceptance and support of the immediate community, especially the Church.

We think it important to emphasize that decision making in serious matters demands a careful examination of what we believe to be true. What we do is a reflection of the convictions we have about life, about God, about man and his relation to the creation. It is impossible to choose a course of action without immediately revealing some of the beliefs that are the foundation stones of our decision making. Consequently, we cannot talk about our response to the dying person without giving serious consideration to what *personhood* means. It is important to ask the question and to challenge our readers to reflect on the matter.

Recent Attempts to Define Personhood

Various attempts made in different disciplines can shed light on what is meant by personhood. For example, the practice of transplanting living body organs has made it imperative to define human death, as the donor must clearly be known to be dead before the tissue is removed. The definition of that state when personal life has ended implies an identification of specific characteristics that indicate the presence of personal existence. As the American philosopher Daniel Maguire suggests:

> Perhaps a case could best illustrate the need for and the nature of a new definition of death. It concerns a twenty-year-old man who suffered a complete shattering of his cerebral cortex in an automobile accident four years previously. Since then only the brain stem has sustained life. All thought and feeling have been erased, and he has not moved a single muscle of his body since the accident. But he is in "excellent health," although he feels no stimulus of any kind, from within or without. Once an angular blond youth of sixteen, he is now a baby-faced "brunette" seemingly ten years old. He is fed through an in-dwelling nasal tube.

Maguire concludes that it "would seem obvious that such a situation requires a declaration of death."[6]

One of the most workable definitions of death has been formulated by the Ad Hoc Committee of the Harvard Medical School. The report outlines the criteria for death in terms of unreceptivity and unresponsivity, no movement or spontaneous breathing, no reflexes, and a flat electroencephalogram over a twenty-four-hour period as confirmation of irreversible coma (excluding cases of hypothermia or central nervous system depressants).[7] A similar definition has been accepted by the Canadian Medical Association.[8]

A large part of the medical professon has come to agree that irreversible cessation of brain function is synonymous with the death of the patient. Some jurisdictions have legislated definitions of death accepting this view. In Manitoba for civil purposes "the death of a person takes place at the time at which irreversible cessation of all that person's brain function occurs" (*Continuing Statutes of Manitoba,* Chapter V — 60, Section 2.1), and a number of states, including Kansas in 1970 and Maryland in 1972, have passed similar legislation.[9]

More recently, the Law Reform Commission of Canada has entered the debate and is recommending the following definition for legislation.

> A person is dead when an irreversible cessation of all that person's brain functions has occurred.
> The cessation of brain functions can be determined by the prolonged absence of spontaneous cardiac and respiratory functions.
> When the determination of the absence of cardiac and respiratory functions is made impossible by the use of artificial means of support, the cessation of the brain functions may be determined by any means recognized by the ordinary standards of current medical practice.[10]

As one might expect, there are many plausible definitions of "brain death." Dr Robert Veatch has researched the subject extensively and comments:

> Most recently in the literature there are those who are beginning to question the adequacy of this notion of brain death, claiming that it already has become old fashioned. They ask why is it that one must identify the entire brain with death; is it not possible that we are really interested only in man's consciousness: in his ability to think, reason, feel, experience, interact with others, and control his body functions consciously? This is crucial in rare cases where the lower brain function might be intact while the cortex, which controls consciousness, is utterly destroyed.[11]

There are various opinions regarding the nature and extent of brain damage that entails the loss of personal existence.

Contributions have also been made by theologians and ethicists. The German Roman Catholic Bernard Häring notes that "a general consensus has been reached that brain death is the end of the earthly history of a human person. With the destruction of the cerebral cortex, the material substratum for any spiritual activity is destroyed; man no longer has the possibility of realizing his personality in freedom and his human history comes to an end."[12] The American author Joseph Fletcher expresses his concern that a more positive statement should be drafted to define personhood. He writes: "In biomedical ethics writers constantly say that we need to explicate humanness or humaneness, what it means to be a truly human being, but they never follow their admission of the need with an actual inventory or profile, no matter how tentatively offered. Yet this is what must be done, or at least attempted."[13] He has suggested minimal criteria by which one could judge whether a living organism is or is not a person. These include minimal intelligence, self-awareness, self-control, a sense of time, of futurity, and of the past, the capability to relate to others, concern for others, communication, control of existence, curiosity, change and changeability, balance of rationality and feeling, idiosyncrasy, and neo-cortical function. Fletcher is obviously attempting a difficult task when he tries to make positive declarations about the human person.

It is not our intention to consider these statements as the basis for any definition of personhood. They serve as illustrations of the debate. It is a serious debate and one that demands a response from the Church. In our approach to the complexities of personhood, we should not expect to achieve a consensus, for there are many diverse currents in theology and ethics. Even though determined efforts have been made in these disciplines to keep pace with scientific and medical discoveries, Dr R.B. Salter observes that the "body of scientific knowledge is growing at a phenomenal rate, certainly much faster than the rate of growth of man's wisdom to manage it."[14] We should reject any attempt to reach a rigid definition of a person or to make decisions easy and routine. Such an approach would degrade and depersonalize decisions which must always be individualized and reached after loving, concerned consideration of the circumstances of each unique person.

What role can theologians play in this ongoing debate? They can, through prayerful study of scripture and the Church's tradition, attempt to formulate what the Christian message means for people today. They can inform our conscience and enable us to reflect on whether or not our actions are loving and compassionate and grounded in what absolutes we can perceive. They can help us act in a meaningful and consistent manner as we try, with responsibility, to avoid the rigidity of religious "law" and to seek, with God's grace, a path that is congruous with our Lord's way.

Man's Relation to God

It would seem fruitless for Christians to search for what is unique in personal human life without first examining man's relation to creation and God. Whatever we say about man will be incomplete until we clarify these relationships. Christians believe that in the beginning God created man in his own "image" and "likeness." He commanded him to "fill the earth and subdue it" and vested in him the responsibility to "rule over the fish in the sea, the birds of heaven, and every living thing that moves upon the earth." (Genesis 1:27, 28. NEB). God has "made him little less than a god, crowning him with glory and honour" (Psalm 8:5. NEB) and has "put all things in subjection beneath his feet" (Hebrews 2:8. NEB).

While we are aware that these statements of faith lend themselves to various interpretations, they are certainly fundamental to the Christian understanding of human nature. Probably the uniqueness of man is most aptly expressed by the idea that he bears within himself the image of God. It is for this reason that men and women claim a respect for their lives and are obliged to offer the same respect to others, a respect which differentiates them from other animate life.

But what does the phrase "image of God" mean? Words such as soul, spirit, or divine spark are often used to describe this likeness. All these refer to that part of God's nature shared with man, by virtue of which man is able to know and love God. It is the link between man and God. These words inspire the imagination and suggest man's experience of God, but we still need to search further to discover the meaning of personhood. How does the "image" manifest itself? What must a person do or be in order for us to recognize the presence of God in that person?

It might be more profitable to an understanding of this problem if we first consider how God manifested himself to us. The basic tenet of the Christian faith is that God became man in Jesus Christ and that, consequently, the nature of God can be known through the life and words of Jesus. He said, "Anyone who has seen me has seen the Father" (John 14:9. NEB). In the life of Jesus, God's infinite self-giving love and compassion is revealed.

The nature and purpose of this revelation is summed up in the First Epistle of John: "For God is love; and his love was disclosed to us in this, that he sent his only Son into the world to bring us life" (4:9. NEB). Christ made the same declaration: "I have come that men may have life, and may have it in all its fullness" (John 10:10. NEB). This life is described in a variety of terms, but possibly the most meaningful is *reconciliation.* In the words of St Paul: "God was in Christ reconciling the world to himself, no longer holding men's misdeeds against them, and... he has entrusted us with the message of reconciliation" (2 Corinthians 5:19. NEB). The loving life and death of Jesus repairs and affirms the relationship, the likeness, between God and man. The ability to partake of this reconciling love displays the "image" we have received and the "good news" we proclaim.

We are not only assured of God's love for us but also of our freedom to respond to it. "You shall know the truth, and the truth will set you free" (John 8:32. NEB). The reconciling act of God is a free gift, and we are capable of responding freely to it. This freedom is another way in which we are like God.

From these considerations it is possible to note certain characteristics that describe the uniqueness of man. He is, above all, a creature able to establish a personal relationship with God. This is possible because man possesses the ability to know God. He also can make responsible moral decisions. Although he is dependent upon the Creator, man has the freedom to share in the renewing love and continuing creative activity of God. The moral theologian G.R. Dunstan succintly states that God "creates man 'in his own image'; that is, with a potential for an identity capable of awareness of God, capable of a freely-willed response to the awakening or call of God, and therefore capable of a consequent likeness with God, of being stamped with his mark, his 'character', his image."[15]

It has become customary in discussions of this kind to speak of the image of God as revealing the sacredness of human life. Some people believe that man possesses a sanctity of life, by virtue of which he may claim a greater degree of respect than other living things. The phrase "sanctity of life" is used widely to describe something unique and special about man, but there are various interpretations of what this word means. Some argue that, because it is inherently sacred, human life must be preserved as long as it endures in any form. Whether one is speaking about comatose life, foetal life, deformed or suffering life, it is asserted that one has no right to make decisions which might endanger its preservation.

Other people believe that such an interpretation leaves no room to consider the quality of life. They argue that it is important for a person to enjoy a certain level of humanity, but that when all possibilities of providing this are gone, attempts to maintain mere biological existence would seem unjustified. Richard A. McCormick, SJ. states the position.

> Life is not a value to be preserved in and for itself. To maintain that would commit us to a form of medical vitalism that makes

no human or Judeo-Christian sense. It is a value to be preserved precisely as a condition for other values, and therefore insofar as these other values remain attainable. Since these other values cluster around and are rooted in human relationships, it seems to follow that life is a value to be preserved only insofar as it contains some potentiality for human relationships. When in human judgment this potentiality is totally absent or would be, because of the condition of the individual, totally subordinated to the mere effort for survival, that life can be said to have achieved its potential.[16]

One of the difficulties of this position lies in clarifying what we mean by quality. In the above quotation, the author refers to "human judgment," and it is at exactly this point that people will add a word of caution. How by human judgment can we safely determine the relative presence or absence of quality in human life?

Edward Keyserlingk has discussed these issues in his valuable paper, *Sanctity of Life or Quality of Life,* recently published by the Law Reform Commission of Canada. Keyserlingk believes that the sanctity of life principle is basic to our society and that its rejection would endanger all human life. Moreover, he says that "to acknowledge and articulate the validity and importance of quality of life concerns need imply in itself no threat to a commitment to the sanctity of life; it need not involve either making the sanctity of life a 'relative' value or positing 'exceptions' to the principle...On the contrary, to acknowledge and attend to quality of life factors... can in fact be a reasonable and necessary expression and defence of the sanctity of life principle itself."[17] Further on, he states that the principle "is *vague and indeterminate but not meaningless.* We do have only a rough, general, 'more or less' idea of what it means. We use in various combinations words such as 'worth', 'value' and 'dignity' when we refer to the principle...it is not meaningless, any more than are the principles of justice or benevolence though they too are indeterminate...the sanctity of life principle does at least 'mean' that life is precious, should be respected and protected, treated with consideration, and is a principle basic to our society."[18] Keyserlingk goes on to assert that "the ethical principle of *respect for persons...,* closely related to that of the sanctity of life, incorporates especially two convictions. The first is that individual persons should be treated as autonomous agents, and the second is that persons with diminished autonomy are entitled to protection by others. That principle and those convictions should always be central in all biomedical decision-making."[19]

It is important to note that man's dignity, worth and sanctity are not conferred on him by other people but rather are gifts from God. Life receives sanctity because of the value God places on it. Human life, having been created by God, belongs to God, and is received by man as a loan. Karl Barth urges:

> Those who handle life as a divine loan will above all treat it with respect....Life does not itself create this respect. The command of God creates respect for it....We may confidently say that the birth of Jesus Christ is the revelation of the command of respect for life. This unmistakably differentiates human life from everything that is done in heaven and earth....And therefore this makes it an object of respect....What matters is not something but someone, the real man before God and among his fellows, his individual psycho-physical existence....Everyone should treat his [own] existence and that of every other human being with respect. For it belongs to God. It is his loan and blessing."[20]

Paul Ramsey expresses it in the same way: "Every human being is a unique, unrepeatable opportunity to praise God. His life is entirely an ordination, a loan, and a stewardship."[21]

Since God is the author of life and man is its trustee, it should be clear that the preservation and nurturing of genuine personal life is the normal obligation of a Christian. The second commandment of Jesus may be paraphrased, "You shall accord the same wholehearted concern and care for your neighbour's life as you give to your own." We are our brother's keeper. All forms of life including animals, being of God's creation, must be respected by man, and our attitude must always proceed from this moral stance. Yet this does not necessarily mean that all forms of life warrant an identical degree of respect. We must judge our response to other people by analyzing the meaning and intent of our actions, testing whether they are based on God's saving love for man and motivated by loving concern for the values and presumed good of the other. We must exercise our moral responsibility conscientiously, taking into account the widest context for our actions and carefully applying the moral principles we have learned from scripture and Christian tradition.

While it is of the utmost importance to be faithful to the moral principles laid down in scripture and tradition, it must be recognized that ethical decisions are often ambiguous, neither absolutely right nor absolutely wrong. We know that during the life of Jesus the traditional moral stance did not always provide him with the opportunity to show his love. On such occasions he went beyond the law. We, too, must be prepared to look at particular situations with the same love. We can do this with confidence because the Christian lives by grace not by rigid law, and God is the ultimate judge of the loving nature of our actions. Our relation to God indicates the unique place of humanity within his total creation. Because we are granted the responsibility to act with God in responding to his creation, we can accord a different level of respect to other forms of life than we must accord to personal life.

Man's Responsibility to God

When we face decisions about those who are dying, it is imperative that we keep in mind those aspects of personhood briefly outlined, using them for general guidance but not as essential criteria. At all times, the image of God must be sought and nurtured and the integrity of the person preserved. In this way we fulfil the commandment to love God and our neighbour. We know that seeking good for our neighbour is no simple task; but if our prime intention is constantly to look for and respond to the image of God in the person under consideration, we believe that we will be acting in the spirit of faith to which God in turn will respond.

It is apparent from the previous discussion that there are two aspects of the person which may conflict. They are his dependence on God and his freedom. Conflict can only be resolved if man acknowledges that he is accountable to God for the exercise of his freedom and that he is a steward of all that has been given in creation, including the gift of life. The new covenant, offered to us by Jesus Christ, establishes that man is the dwelling place of the Holy Spirit and permits him to act for God, to be a "co-creator" with him. Man is the agent through whom God continues his work of creation in this world. Bernard Häring puts this case strongly. He writes:

> Belief in one God, Creator of all things, is a call to co-responsibility....The Incarnation establishes a new relationship between man and the ongoing creation; it testifies to God's constant

presence to man through his work....Revelation has an eschatological orientation. While gratefully recollecting all past efforts, it calls for openness to the here and now and for readiness in setting out for new horizons....a theology for the pilgrim situation of man inspires hope and demands responsibility for the future....The doctrine of the Incarnation and Redemption guarantees man (especially the physician) full freedom in the service of his fellow-man to the best of his ability without being hemmed in by taboos. It likewise safeguards the dignity of the human person in a perspective of the total vocation of man.[22]

In other words, we have to accept in the light of reality the freedom that modern technology gives, always remembering our relation to our Creator and Redeemer. "Christ set us free, to be free men" (Galatians 5:1. NEB).

The freedom to exercise our co-responsibility with God concerning decisions about sickness, life and death, is given to the fellowship of those who care — physicians and other health-professionals, family and patient — and to reject this responsibility and freedom is to deny the stewardship with which we are entrusted. For God expects us to engage in creative decision making, fulfilling our personhood and the image of God within us, by sharing this responsibility.

Advances in technology have given us increasing control over our environment and our fate, with enormous and obvious benefits. They also bring unavoidable moral and ethical problems. Our values are continually evolving, and we should question whether values established in the past about man and society are still applicable to the new challenges and problems that confront us today.

While the mind functions and relationships with God and other persons are possible, we are without question dealing with genuine personal life. Is it valid to ask whether or not there are situations in which life no longer has personal values that justify continued medical life support? We must distinguish between the preservation of life with no potential for maintaining personal existence and the preservation of life with impaired and restricted personal qualities. Indeed, Keyserlingk argues that in some cases the quality of the patient's life may be so damaged that his biological life is not of the same value and that treatment could be a violation of that life's sanctity.[23]

Can man's freedom include decisions, reached while still rational, concerning his death and those situations in which he no longer wishes his life to be preserved? Co-responsibility suggests that we are called to play an important role in shaping our lives and affecting our destiny. We believe this responsibility extends to our dying and to deciding under what circumstances we ought to cling to life. Jesus was very decisive on this point. He talked openly with his disciples about his death and made clear that he felt a genuine responsibility for all his actions, including his dying.

Doctors are sometimes accused of "playing God" as they exercise their responsibility to make decisions about the dying person. By this is meant an arrogant, overbearing independence and refusal to accept the restraint and guidance which human dependence on God requires. For the vast majority of doctors, this is an unjust and unwarranted accusation, and it maligns the integrity of the medical profession. Decisiveness is *not* the same as unrestrained autonomy. Even as Christians are obliged to be co-responsible with God in decisions which affect his creation, so doctors also are called upon to "play God's part" as they pursue their professional responsibility in the service of their patients. They are trained to accept the responsibility of making life and death decisions and do so every day. Their patients properly expect this and trust the medical profession to decide justly and honestly.

We should all be concerned with this area of personal responsibility and consider not only the quality of our living, but also the quality of our dying. When we are rational, our responsibility to participate in decisions concerning our own death is paramount. Families may do a grave injustice to a dying person by withholding information about terminal illness. Such a protective sentiment, intended as an act of love, deprives the patient of the chance to participate personally and consciously in the climax of his life. The conspiracy of silence and denial, intended to ease the patient, may fail to do so and, indeed, may frighten those whose greatest need at this unique stage of their lives is for genuine candour.

Dr David Skelton has worked extensively with terminal patients in the Palliative Care Unit of St Boniface Hospital, Winnipeg. He makes the following observations:

> I was recently interrogated by two medical students after an interview with a dying patient in which her searching questions had been answered honestly and as gently as possible. "When does it become easy to tell such a patient that she is likely to die?" asked one of them who only a few minutes before had been literally moved to tears at the patient's bedside. The day in

which such an interaction fails to evoke pain within the attendant is, I believe, the day in which he should retire from the field of health care. It should never become merely a ritualistic action devoid of feeling and commitment. We must constantly be on guard lest our fear of self-inflicted pain in these circumstances should inhibit or curtail our availability and our consistently honest interaction with the dying individual.

Who is the ideal person to do the telling? In my opinion anyone asked by the patient can undertake this responsibility, given that they know the answers and can handle the process of information exchange. There is no place here for guess work or assumption; no attempt to maintain one's personal or professional image at the expense of total honesty can be allowed. Dying patients frequently choose the time and the person for questions of information with great care, and such questioning may have required great courage on their part. The fact that they do not always choose one particular person or profession should not inhibit the vital flow of communication that is being requested.

Great sensitivity is required of the attendants in this situation; we require ability not only to listen, but to hear — not only to respond, but to feel. It is frequently the unasked questions that require answers most urgently, and these can only be recognized through patience, trust, and true empathy. It is my opinion that sympathy is often a destructive response, whereas empathy — a compassionate willingness to share all that we can of the other's problem — can be the foundation for great healing.[24]

It is our belief that this sharing expresses our responsibility to God and our fellow man.

Summary

This section of the report has not been designed to give specific answers to the problems associated with the terminally ill, but rather to provide a Christian stance from which we may properly approach the issues. It would be presumptuous of us to search for definitions which could put an end to this debate. It is far more important that we clarify our attitudes and beliefs about man and his relationship with God in order to establish the right framework in which to ask the right questions, and by the grace of God to reach those particular decisions which affect the unique situations of individual persons. It is also important that we engage in this task with the understanding that God wishes us to undertake this responsibility. We must neither overestimate our ability nor underrate our responsibility. It is with this kind of humility and courage that we can examine the complex moral, social, and legal issues which have arisen around dying in recent times.

2
Decisions about Life and Death

We now turn to consider those situations in which it is necessary to decide whether or not to preserve life. They involve people who are suffering from incurable disease or critical injury or who are born with gross and uncorrectable defects. In most areas of the world such questions do not arise because there are not enough medical resources even to care for those who can be cured, and most sick persons perforce remain untreated. Decisions of this kind are the result of medical progress in affluent countries with highly developed health systems. Scientific advances, as they bear on individual circumstances, demand answers which it is irresponsible to evade. In fact, not to decide is an arbitrary and potentially devastating decision by default.[1] For instance treatment may be continued, to the patient's detriment.

The right to life stems from the undeniable fact that life is "the fundamental context in which all other goods which God has given man, must be exercised."[2] Since dying is the final stage of life on earth for each of us, one may conclude that a person has the moral right to refuse treatment under some circumstances, even though this may result in death, and also the right to have some influence on and decision about the way in which he dies. Medical technology can now significantly affect the mode and time of death, and to this extent has put dying into the area of human choice. The exercise of this choice, when used to make death as easy and gentle as possible and when motivated by the good of the patient, has been called *euthanasia.* Although this word has had a broad meaning, today it commonly refers to "mercy killing."

Explanation of Terms

Voluntary and Involuntary Euthanasia — If the individual concerned is rational, and in the legal sense competent, the choice of ceasing the struggle to live may be reached jointly by the patient and the medical attendants. This has been called voluntary euthanasia. If, on the other hand, the patient is comatose, otherwise irrational, or legally incompetent, the decision may be reached by agreement between the patient's immediate family or legal guardian (the patient's surrogates) and the medical attendants. Because the patient is unable to take part in the decision, this may be termed involuntary euthanasia. An exception, however, arises in the case of legal minors who are rational and have reached the age of comprehension. Since they are able to know and reason about their medical condition, the preservation of their autonomy requires that they be as fully involved in the decision as the legally competent patient and moves the decision into the voluntary category.

Passive and Active Euthanasia — It has been usual to distinguish between two kinds of euthanasia, passive and active. Both voluntary and involuntary euthanasia can be either passive or active. Passive euthanasia has been considered to mean the omission of medical treatment when it is expected that the patient will die without such treatment. It thus includes:

(1) The decision not to begin life-preserving treatment, for example, not to administer antibiotics to a patient with terminal cancer;

(2) the decision to stop treatment already begun, for example, to terminate a programme of kidney dialysis or courses of chemotherapy for cancer.

However, many would say that such decisions do not involve euthanasia at all but merely good medical practice when it is recognized that the treatment is not beneficial and when the patient is allowed to die while receiving care to maintain comfort.

It has been customary also to include in passive euthanasia the administration of treatment to relieve severe pain, usually drugs that may have the unintended but possible consequence of causing or hastening death which is already near. However, because death is then not intentional, this also is not euthanasia in any real sense, but rather purely symptomatic and palliative treatment for the patient's benefit. Consequently some argue that the term *passive euthanasia* should be dropped.

Active euthanasia means the commission of a positive act to end the patient's life — typically a medically administered lethal injection but sometimes action by distraught relatives. This, if prompted by a genuine concern for the patient's perceived good, is indeed mercy killing, perhaps performed at the patient's request; it should not necessarily be considered wanton or reckless disregard for life. Whether or not this action is morally justifiable, and what consequences might flow from it, will be discussed later. Discontinuing the use of medical apparatus thought to be essential for continued life is usually considered passive euthanasia. An example is disconnecting a respirator. It has been argued however that *once instituted* the cessation of such life-support apparatus is as much a positive act as a lethal injection; this is in contradistinction to a decision *not to begin* its use. The former is an act of commission, the latter of omission. This argument suggests that disconnecting a respirator or similar apparatus is equivalent to active euthanasia. Most doctors would not agree with this conclusion, because a lethal injection is a direct interference with nature whereas disconnecting a respirator allows the patient to live or die as a natural consequence of his disease or injury. The Clinical Care Committee of the Massachusetts General Hospital has described turning off a respirator as a definite act of commission.[3] This discussion suggests that the distinction between active and passive euthanasia is not always sharply evident. Rather than using these adjectives, it might then be more useful to distinguish euthanasia by commission from euthanasia by omission. We may summarize this description of euthanasia as follows: in euthanasia by commission (active), the person who acts determines the outcome; in euthanasia by omission (passive), the illness is left to take its course, uninfluenced by treatment, and the patient may live or die.

Ordinary and Extraordinary Treatment — Consideration must also be given to the distinction between "ordinary" and "extraordinary" (or heroic) treatment. Briefly, treatment is ordinary when it is easily available, gives reasonable hope of success, and is acceptable to the patient and / or the family. To be ordinary, the treatment must be customary in the institution or community and in the circumstances in which a particular patient finds himself. Ordinary treatment does not entail grave hardship to the patient. When these conditions are not fulfilled, the treatment may be considered extraordinary. A particular mode of treatment may be ordinary or extraordinary, depending upon the circumstances. For example, antibiotics, which are usually ordinary and indeed mandatory, become extraordinary when given to prolong life briefly in a patient who is dying of cancer, unless they are indicated for the relief of distressing symptoms. However, yesterday's heroic efforts often become today's routine procedures.[4]

Theological and Moral Reflections on Euthanasia

What spiritual insights can be found to illuminate our present capability to influence the process of dying? In many cases continued treatment does no more than prolong this process, and the end can be foreseen in the near future. Treatment itself may cause physical and mental suffering,* and when the prospect of cure begins to recede, the rationale of persisting with treatment is weakened. Some forms of treatment may cause complications that make the patient more sick or even precipitate death. When faced with the decision whether or not to stop treatment, those concerned must consider the favourable effect to be reasonably expected, the probable duration of life, and the value of that life as seen by the patient, his immediate associates, and his doctor. These factors must be weighed against the risks of serious complications and the suffering inherent in the treatment itself.

It is necessary to give some explanation of the word *hopeless* in the medical context. There are, of course, clinical signs which indicate, without any significant shadow of doubt, that death is imminent. Apart from this, no doctor can be absolutely positive that a particular patient will die as a result of his disease or injury. It can sometimes be stated that no patient with a given set of clinical findings has ever been known to survive. More often a doctor can state that, from his own experience, the experience of the hospital in which the patient is treated, or experience reported in the medical literature, it is his opinion that the chances of survival are minimal. Doctors can never be absolutely dogmatic, for patients may show as much variability in dying as in the rest of life. In a given case the doctor can only say that, to the best of his belief, knowledge, and experience, survival is extremely improbable and sometimes unprecedented. The chance of survival is then so remote that it would be folly to let it influence decisions. Lack of absolute certainty is part of the dilemma confronting the doctor concerned with the apparently dying patient and is inevitable in the practice of medicine. The objection that even a minimal

---

*Suffering in general is discussed in Part III — ''Facing Pain and Suffering.''

chance of survival compels us to try to preserve life at any cost, shows a failure to recognize the suffering which will be inflicted on many to uncertain purpose. There is no way to identify in advance any benefit to the few. Another example of the predicaments facing doctors is the equal difficulty in foretelling, except in the broadest of terms, the length of life remaining for a given patient.

It follows from the earlier discussion that respect for life requires its preservation and protection as the norm. Nevertheless, if we turn to God, we may come to the conviction that there are exceptions to this norm. We think that in our exercise of co-responsibility under God, we must try to discern when such exceptions occur. Once such a conclusion is reached we believe we are morally bound to follow the necessary course. It is not irresponsible, under some circumstances, to desire that one's own life or that of a loved relative should not be prolonged. In these decisions, the Christian remembers that death is not essentially evil. Indeed, leaving a tired and painful body to enter a closer relationship with God may be good, provided one has become reconciled with God and with those around one. In our view, respect for the life and values of a person may, in some circumstances, be shown only by refusing to prolong his life. In this way, the patient's highest good may be attained. Reflecting on the extremes of medical technology Karl Barth claims that

> the question also arises whether this kind of artificial prolongation of life does not amount to human arrogance...whether the fulfillment of medical duty does not threaten to become fanaticism, reason folly and the required assisting of human life a forbidden torturing of it....a doctor might have to recoil from this prolongation of life....it may well be that in this special sphere we do have a kind of exceptional case....it is a question of the respect which may be claimed by even the dying life.[5]

While we must be concerned to avoid arbitrary and subjective decisions, to specify precisely the conditions under which aggressive treatment should be stopped would put us at odds with life. We must proceed from the broad principles of respect for life and love of neighbour and, under the guidance of the Holy Spirit, thread our way through the choice of options which medical capability has brought. Instead of decrying the consequent complexity and ambiguity, we have the responsibility to reach individualized decisions, insisting that they be made from a theological and moral perspective and not solely from the scientific and technical point of view.

It is apparent that the great majority of the medical profession believes there is a sharp, moral distinction between passive and active euthanasia. Surveys have indicated that most doctors, with a wide range of religious beliefs, support the position that it is morally correct not to prolong life in appropriate circumstances, and they will consequently withdraw or not institute treatment, so allowing death to occur. Conversely, very few doctors believe that active euthanasia is ever justified, and hardly any would consider practising it.[6]

The House of Delegates of the American Medical Association in December 1973 adopted the following statement.

> The intentional termination of life of one human being by another — mercy killing — is contrary to that for which the medical profession stands and is contrary to the policy of the American Medical Association. The cessation of the employment of extraordinary means to prolong the life of the body when there is irrefutable evidence that biological death is imminent is the decision of the patient and / or his immediate family. The advice and judgment of the physician should be freely available to the patient and / or his immediate family.[7]

However, the philosopher James Rachels has put the following argument for equating active and passive euthanasia on moral grounds. If treatment is simply withheld, it may take longer for the terminal patient to die, and so he may suffer more than if direct action were taken. This is contrary to the humanitarian attitude which prompts the decision not to prolong life. Direct action, being quick and painless, may be more humane. In his view, a doctor's moral position may be identical whether, for humane reasons, he allows a patient to die or whether, for the same reasons, he administers a lethal injection. The intended effect is the same in each case. If the doctor's judgment was incorrect and in fact the patient's condition was curable, the decision to end life would be just as blameworthy whichever method was used. Equally, if the decision was correct, the approach used would not of itself be important.[8] Paul Ramsey, among others, has argued to the contrary.

> The difference between only *caring for the dying*, and *acts of euthanasia* is not a choice between indirectly and directly willing

and doing something. It is rather the important choice between doing something and doing nothing, or (better said) ceasing to do something that was begun i.e. life sustaining treatment, in order to do something that is better because now more fitting. In omission no human agent causes the patient's death, directly or indirectly. He dies his own death from causes that it is no longer merciful or reasonable to fight by means of possible medical interventions.... In any case, doing something or omitting something in order to do something else, are different sorts of acts. To do or not to do something may, then, be subject to different moral evaluations.[9]

American philosopher Hans Jonas, considering the morality of complying with the patient's right to discontinue life support, asserts that it is entirely fallacious in this case to "equate desisting with doing, thus permitting to die with killing."[10]

The reason for the medical profession's rejection of active euthanasia is summed up in the phrase "contrary to that for which the medical profession stands." Doctors are trained to diagnose and treat disease and to oppose death. This can lead to an inability to recognize that treatment in some circumstances is doomed to failure and that death cannot be prevented. The medical profession has long ago moved from the position that it was concerned only with the physical ills of the body and now recognizes an equal responsibility to treat diseases of the mind. Because body and mind are closely interwoven, disease of the one has profound effects on the other. Is it too idealistic to suggest that a doctor's concern should not be confined to the body and mind but should comprehend the patient's entire person? Should not the doctor's role include the health of the spirit as well as the health of the mind and body? Dr Eric Cassell, professor of public health at Cornell University Medical College, has stated this position in different terms.

I believe that the function of medicine is to preserve autonomy and that preservation of life is subservient to the primary goal.... If the preservation of autonomy is the goal of medicine, then one must do everything possible to maintain the integrity of the person in the face of death.[11]

These considerations have led some to argue that the highest interest of the patient as a complete entity and the preservation of his integrity, autonomy, and values, may in occasional circumstances justify the use of active euthanasia as the most compassionate and moral way to achieve these ends. They argue that such a course of action might be compatible with respect for life and seeking our neighbour's good.

However, those who work in palliative care units or hospices realize that requests by dying patients for active euthanasia are almost invariably precipitated by the need for improved management of symptoms. The symptomatic distress is often pain but may be breathlessness, nausea, vomiting, diarrhoea, or offensive discharges. If these symptoms are adequately ameliorated, patients will no longer ask that their lives be actively terminated. Cicely Saunders notes,

> If you relieve a patient's pain and if you can make him feel like a wanted person — which he is, then you are not going to be asked about euthanasia.... Euthanasia is an admission of defeat (failure of management), and a totally negative approach. One should be working to see that it is not needed.[12]

We must recognize that strong feelings are aroused by discussion of this subject but it deserves careful consideration, especially by those who believe that death is not the ultimate evil.

Regarding the distinction between ordinary and extraordinary care, Pope Pius XII made the following comments in an allocation delivered to a congress of anaesthetists in November 1957.

> But normally one is held to use only ordinary means — according to circumstances of persons, places, times, and culture — that is to say, means that do not involve any grave burden for oneself or another. A more strict obligation would be too burdensome for most men and would render the attainment of the higher, more important good too difficult. Life, health, all temporal activities are in fact subordinated to spiritual ends. On the other hand, one is not forbidden to take more than the strictly necessary steps to preserve life and health, as long as he does not fail in some more serious duty....
>
> Consequently, if it appears that the attempt at resuscitation constitutes in reality such a burden for the family that one cannot in all conscience impose it upon them, they can lawfully insist that the doctor should discontinue these attempts, and the doctor can lawfully comply.[13]

The former Archbishop of Canterbury, Dr Coggan, shared the same concern in his Edwin Stevens Lecture delivered in December

1976. Citing a commentary made on the Papal Allocution in *Decisions About Life and Death,* he noted:

> The answer given in the Allocution was based on the distinction, already drawn by Roman Catholic moralists, between "ordinary" and "extraordinary" medical or surgical procedures. "Ordinary" in this context does not mean what a medical man would regard as "normal" treatment: it means whatever a patient can obtain and undergo without thereby imposing an excessive burden on himself or others. Thus "extraordinary" treatment has been defined as whatever here and now is very costly or very unusual or very painful or very difficult or very dangerous, or if the good effects that can be expected from its use are not proportionate to the difficulty and inconvenience that are entailed.[14]

Father R.A. McCormick, S.J., as mentioned before, has explored these issues. He argues that the meaning of life (the higher, more important good) is seriously jeopardized when undue and unending effort must go into its maintenance (too difficult). If the quality of the life preserved is painful, deprived, and oppressive, this establishes the means required as extraordinary, because the potential for growth in love of God and neighbour would no longer function as the purpose and meaning of the individual's life, and mere existence would become the ultimate value. There comes a point where an individual's condition itself negates any truly personal potential and the best treatment is no treatment. For McCormick life is a value to be preserved, not in and for itself but as a condition for other values rooted in human relationships, and only so far as these values remain attainable. When in human judgment the potential for personal relationships is totally subordinated to the mere effort for survival, that life can be said to have no further potential. Yet because another's capacity for relationships is a matter of human judgment and mistakes will be made, we must proceed with great humility, caution, and tentativeness, tilting our judgment on the side of life.[15]

Let us now see if these reflections help us in the care of three types of patients for whom decisions about prolonging life may be required. In many of these cases a therapeutic stage is reached when the line between life and death coincides with that between continuation and cessation of treatment; in others the treatment ceases to ameliorate the illness, let alone cure it. At this point it is necessary to use some medical terminology to insure clarity and avoid misunderstanding.

The Rational, Terminally-Ill Patient

The definition of *terminal* is arbitrary and may be thought of in terms of a few months. A patient with a terminal illness may foresee the end as clearly as his medical attendants. He may be stricken with advanced cancer or with end-stage damage to the heart, lungs, or other vital organs. A patient in this group may see no further value in prolonging his life span, either to himself or to those around him. He may then express a deliberate and consistent request that life-preserving treatment be discontinued, a request with which the family may or may not agree. At this stage, continued treatment may be seen by the patient and the doctor as nothing more than the infliction of an injury. Ought the doctor to comply with the request and allow death to occur? Love of neighbour may suggest that he should.

The patient with end-stage kidney disease is in a rather different position, because life can now be maintained for long periods by kidney dialysis. However, the health of some dialysis patients is poor, and unless he receives a kidney transplant, the patient faces a never-ending program of dialysis on a thrice-weekly basis. The usual practice to enable dialysis to be undertaken is to create an artificial connection between a medium-sized artery and vein by a minor operation. At each session of dialysis, large needles are inserted into the blood vessels close to this "shunt" to pass blood into the machine and then return it to the body. The patient must be connected to the machine for several hours. The blood vessels may gradually deteriorate so that new shunts need to be fashioned, perhaps every two years. Unfortunate complications may occur in the shunt: blood may clot and block it, and infection and disruption of the blood vessels may occur. When this happens, immediate operative correction is required. The prospect of interminable dependence on the dialysis machine, punctuated by a succession of operations (though these are minor), may become unbearable for a few patients.

There is no question that one has the legal right to refuse treatment, even if the refusal will result in death. Does one have the same right on moral grounds in some circumstances, or is one morally obligated to continue to live as long as possible? The patient may have family or public responsibilities which restrict freedom of choice. Before choosing, he must know the prognosis of his illness and think through the possible alternative courses of action. However, he cannot act on his decision without the compliance of those caring for him. It is the doctor's duty to enable a decision to be made on the basis of "informed consent." The patient has the right to open and truthful discussion before exercising his right to refuse treatment, and hence to risk almost certain death. One may well believe that this latter right is morally justified when the patient who is terminally ill or critically injured concludes that his death has become of more value to himself and his family than his continued life.

The Patient in Irreversible Coma

There are many patients in irreversible coma for whom decisions about the preservation of life are required. The state of the patient may be the result of disease but is frequently due to violent injury, particularly from motor vehicle accidents. Irreversible coma is sometimes called brain death. Although there is permanent loss of brain function, other physiological processes of the body, such as digestion or urinary secretion, continue spontaneously or are maintained by artificial means, the respirator being the prime example. In this sense, the patient is not in a terminal state, but by definition, he is completely out of contact with his environment and is no longer able to make decisions. The doctor and the family together must decide on the patient's behalf.

If life is maintained only by a respirator, is it genuine personal life or simply biological or "technical" life? Certainly, the life still present is human. The individual is of human stock and the body contains living organs which can be transplanted and function in other human patients. Although human life still exists, can this patient any longer be considered a person when the brain is dead and the anatomical basis of personality has been destroyed? If one accepts that death of the brain is synonymous with death of the person, then turning off the respirator would only be an admission that death has already occurred, and this is not euthanasia in any true sense. It may well be argued that to preserve life in such a patient, so far from showing respect for life, is rather an indignity and a mark of disrespect to the memory of the person that the patient once was. A right to die can be asserted in defence of the past dignity of the person, which is degraded by such continuing "survival."[16] These considerations are part of the frequently expressed wish for "death with dignity."

Pope Pius XII stated that "when deep unconsciousness is judged to be permanent, extraordinary means to maintain life are not obligatory. They can be terminated and the patient allowed to die."[17] There is thus convincing support from the medical, ethical, humanitarian, and religious points of view for the position that irreversible coma is sufficient reason to terminate life-preserving treatment. Sometimes the family of the patient may first raise the question whether it is appropriate to discontinue treatment. More often the doctor, because of his knowledge and experience, will consider this option first. He must then explain the situation to the family and seek their concurrence. The final decision must be taken jointly.

The situation is different when all physiological processes, except those of the brain are maintained spontaneously and a respirator or other artificial support is not required for continued survival. This was the case with Karen Quinlan. In April 1975 this young girl took an overdose of drugs which, combined with an intake of alcohol, rendered her comatose, and all tests indicated that the coma was irreversible. A respirator was used to breathe for her, and her doctors considered that life would cease if the use of the respirator was ended. Her father, believing that further treatment was not warranted, obtained legal authority for the respirator to be turned off. When this was done, the patient resumed spontaneous breathing. Life and the coma continued. Another instance of this situation might be a patient who has sustained a severe stroke. As long as the patient is given fluids, nourishment, and regular nursing care — in fact, ordinary treatment — he may survive for weeks, months, or even years, until other physiological processes of the body (such as those of the heart, lungs, and kidneys) fail, often as the result of infection. Clearly, these patients do not suffer, though their loving families do. No doubt it would generally be agreed that administering antibiotics for infection, or treating other complications to prolong such a patient's survival, would constitute extraordinary treatment and would be inappropriate.

These patients do not fulfil the criteria of brain death set out by the Committee of the Harvard Medical School, because spontaneous respiration continues,[18] but the cerebral cortex is dead, as shown by clinical signs and the electroencephalogram. In this situation, the following questions may be raised, and they require answers.

(1) In the particular circumstances of this patient, does treatment usually considered "ordinary" in effect become "extraordinary" in view of the pointless prolongation of purely biological life? Should even the provisions of fluids and nourishment, administered by stomach tube or intravenously, be considered extraordinary and therefore be discontinued?

(2) To avoid slow physical deterioration and the prolonged misery of the family, would some form of active euthanasia be compatible with compassion for the patient and family, and with respect for the past life and dignity of the patient?

The Newborn Infant with Gross and Uncorrectable Defects

This group of patients, hitherto small in number, has become increasingly numerous with the development of intensive care nurseries. Moreover, their treatment arouses even greater concern in society at large than that of the previous two groups. Hence, we shall examine the issues at length and in detail.

We must bear two important factors in mind. The first is that all children at birth lack responsibility and self-determination. The characteristics of personhood are only awakened by a process of social interaction, usually starting with the parents. Without such interaction, the development of every child would be limited. The potential for the development of personal characteristics is realized as the intellectual functions of the brain develop. Children at birth are granted the same value and rights as adults precisely because of their potential as persons. Unhappily, some of our fellows are born with varying degrees of faulty development of the brain cortex, and their personal development is therefore limited. In some respects they remain in the state from which all infants start to develop and which normally is temporary.[19] When intellectual function is impaired, these persons are called mentally retarded.

Infants may also sustain brain damage during birth, sometimes the result of injuries during delivery but more often caused by interference with the cerebral circulation. The latter deprives the brain of vital oxygen in varying degrees (cerebral anoxia). In either case, these children may show varying grades of mental retardation and physical disability (cerebral palsy, spasticity).

It cannot, however, be asserted too strongly that, so long as such individuals might attain a minimal degree of self-determination or can engage in some social interaction, they are indeed persons, even though they lack the potential to reach the level of personal development open to those of us who are not so afflicted. A number of such retarded infants are born with additional abnormalities which, if uncorrected, will lead to death. To an increasing degree, these associated abnormalities are becoming surgically correctable, often with small risk and with excellent prospects of success. An example is the infant with Down's Syndrome who also has a congenital obstruction of the intestinal tract. Having accepted the argument that retarded infants are indeed possessed of personhood, one is morally bound to afford them the necessary surgical aid to allow continued life. It is clear that neither all parents nor all doctors accept this imperative, and a number of infants with correctable intestinal obstruction are not treated and die, for the sole reason that they have Down's Syndrome.[20] We believe that this is morally wrong.

A second factor is the progress that has been achieved in recent years in the training of retarded children who often have additional physical handicaps. Infants once considered to be totally and permanently defective in mental capacity now are increasingly found to be trainable, so that they can function and relate to others, at least at a basic level. Moreover, it is now recognized that it is very difficult to predict in early life which infants are trainable and what level of mental development such training may achieve. Even the professional in this field has not infrequently been proved wrong, in a pessimistic early prognosis, by the unexpected and surprisingly encouraging development of a retarded child.[21] Unfortunately, a large part of the medical profession remains unaware of the advances in these therapeutic techniques. Unless he has this knowledge, a doctor should be very hesitant to come to final decisions about retarded children.

The Church in every generation has recognized its duty to protect and support the weak and disadvantaged. It is a Christian ethic that the strong must support and aid the weak and helpless even at the cost of the strong. Hence the mandate to serve infants with less than full potential. With these considerations firmly in mind, let us consider two examples of congenital disease in which decisions are exceedingly complex and possibly controversial.

First, there is a group of defects of the spinal cord generally comprehended by the terms "myelomeningocoele" or "open spina bifida." In this condition, the coverings of the cord are incomplete so that there is an opening in the back through which the cord and nerve roots bulge outwards. These are either exposed or covered only by a tenuous membrane which is easily injured, infected, and desiccated. The infant suffers partial to total paralysis of the legs, incontinence of bowel and bladder, severe spinal deformities, actual or potential hydrocephaly, and often mental retardation in varying degrees. The complications of kidney damage, leg deformities, and ocular derangements frequently supervene. The higher the level of the defect in the back, the more severe are its effects.

Treatment usually involves a succession of operations. If there is any movement in the legs, operation is required immediately after birth to preserve this motor function and to prevent infection. Subsequently operations for the correction of hydrocephaly and orthopaedic deformities in the legs and back are often necessary as well as additional operations to mitigate incontinence, prevent kidney infection, and control eye complications. A treatment program of this nature enables many such children to survive. However, nearly all survivors are crippled, leading a wheel chair life or requiring braces and crutches. Most remain incontinent, and many have various levels of mental retardation. While treatment can prolong life, it often does little to reduce disability and suffering,[22] but without it most of these children decline slowly in the months following birth and die within a year, despite the best of supportive and nursing care.[23]

Experience (e.g. at Cambridge, England) indicates that, in about half of those children who are treated and survive, disability is occasionally minimal or more often moderate. In the other half it is severe or very severe.[24] Selection of those infants who will derive significant benefit from treatment is difficult, but is the practice of many medical teams who wish to avoid embarking on a course of treatment that is not in the infant's best interest and that might then be regarded as the infliction of additional injury. Selection may be based on the level of the defect and the negative factors of complete paralysis of the legs and of hydrocephaly at birth.[25] However, because there are at present no infallible criteria for determining potential at birth, other medical teams operate on all infants with myelomeningocele to close the defect and relieve the hydrocephaly.[26]

Secondly, with the advent of intensive care nurseries, many premature infants with very low birth weights are now enabled to live when formerly their outlook was virtually hopeless. Such infants are born with immature lungs and often need respirator support or care in incubators with an enriched oxygen atmosphere for many days. Unfortunately, high concentrations of oxygen administered over long periods may seriously damage the lungs. In the extreme case, it may become impossible for the infant to continue to live without added oxygen. Even short of this, the time may come when it is necessary to consider whether the lung damage is permanent and of such severity that the infant will be a respiratory cripple. From this consideration will stem a decision whether or not to continue respirator support.

Myelomeningocoele and prematurity are just two examples of an increasing number of disease states in the newborn infant which involve decisions having moral and ethical, as well as medical, implications.[27] However, there are other uncommon abnormalities in the newborn which are no less tragic but about which decision is less difficult to reach and is less likely to be controversial. Among these are infants in whom there is complete failure of the cerebral cortex to develop, such as cerebral agenesis and anencephaly. Beyond all question, these infants have no potential whatever to enter the world of mankind; they will forever be dependent on others for every function of living and will never gain the slightest capacity for social interaction. Can we recognize as meaningful an entity which lacks the neurological basis of conscious life?[28] Many of these infants are stillborn: if they are born living and the gross anomaly of the head is readily apparent, it would generally be agreed that efforts to initiate breathing should not be made. If the infant breathes spontaneously, it usually dies within hours or days of birth, but this is not invariably the case. With ordinary nursing care, the infant may thrive and live for several weeks. The usual practice is not to place the infant on a regular program of feeding, but only to give sugar and water when it appears hungry. However, some of these infants cannot swallow, and in any case such administration of fluids only serves to prolong the intended progress to death which results from inadequate nutrition, insufficient fluids, and perhaps infection. While the decision not to preserve life would likely be generally accepted, the means of attaining the end seem inhumane and unmerciful. Would active euthanasia be more compassionate? The alternative is to support them to the best of our ability for their short lives.

There are some genetic disorders which bear a similarity to what has just been discussed. Among them are Trisomy D (13) and E (18). In these conditions, there are multiple physical defects and profound mental retardation. They occur once in every 3,000 to 5,000 live births. Most of these newborns die in infancy and survival beyond one year is exceptional. They need only regular nursing care and no treatment has any effect on the course of the disease. It is a mercy that they do not appear to suffer and that death releases them soon and gently. These conditions are mentioned here as examples of newborn disease in which it would likely be generally accepted that attempts to prolong life are inappropriate.

These trisomy states must be totally distinguished from Trisomy G (21). This condition, also known as Down's Syndrome, is much more frequent, and the outlook is radically different. Many of these infants are only moderately retarded and have a life expectancy of many years. Such children can usually live at home with their families, enjoying a restricted and protected, but relatively normal and happy life. When they become adolescents and adults, they can often achieve a measure of independence. Though their intellect does not develop as fully, yet they are persons, and any associated physical defects, which threaten life, should be corrected so that they can realize their potential to the greatest degree possible.

What spiritual help and guidance can we find in those situations where the newborn's defects are severe? All will feel the utmost compassion for the infant, the parents, and those charged with medical care, as they confront the decision whether or not to preserve life. Although, in some instances, the decision may be reached readily and with general agreement, far more often the predicament is desperate and no solution is satisfactory. The temptation to delay decision is strong, in the hopes that the infant will contract an infection which, without treatment, will cause rapid and merciful death. The doctor, having assessed the infant in the light of those factors which indicate the likely results both with and without treatment, has to explain the alternatives to the parents as fully but as simply as possible, so that they can reach an informed opinion. Exercising their responsibility together, parents and doctors must seek to discern the course which appears to be for the infant's greatest good. Since the clinical condition of such infants is so variable, we must expect and tolerate much latitude in decision.[29] We do not know how often parents and doctors will make just decisions for the infant. Some argue that no one is better placed to do so, considering their intimate knowledge of the unique situation and the reality that the decision is often urgent. Others suggest there is need for more objective decision making — for instance, by a tribunal of persons not involved with the patient. When there is real doubt, they should choose to preserve life. The family's pastor or the hospital chaplain can help the parents as they wrestle with the alternatives, and it is through him that the Church can express consolation and support. The parents must be helped to live with the decision afterwards, so that they are neither destroyed by guilt if they refuse treatment nor overburdened by care if the child continues to live. When we know that the decision has been reached responsibly, not hurriedly, and with real soul-searching, we think the Church should accept it, even though some individual Christians may doubt its wisdom. Certainly, no one who has not been personally involved in such a situation, can fully understand the agony involved in making these decisions.

Possible Consequences of Active Euthanasia

Some would claim that active euthanasia might be appropriate, compassionate, moral, and theologically justified for two types of patient: the individual in irreversible coma who is breathing spontaneously and the newborn infant in whom the cerebral cortex has totally failed to develop. Both types lead only a biological existence, and personhood has died or never existed. Their tragedy puts severe strain on their families and the staff who care for them. Human life, but not personhood, lingers on until the functions of other body organs fail, often as a result of infection. Thus some suggest that the impasse could be swiftly and humanely ended by a lethal injection.

It has been argued that the exercise of this option would brutalize those who committed it, even though undertaken with the purest of motives. Certainly the action would entail stress for the doctor involved and, to a lesser degree, for other members of the staff who had been caring for the patient, even though all believed it to be the lesser of two evils. Emotional trauma, combined with traditional religious and philosophical doubts, would certainly deter many doctors from this course and would, at the very least, demand rigorous soul-searching and medical consultation at the highest level before the action was undertaken. Long survival of the patients we have described is unusual and the option of active euthanasia would therefore arise infrequently. However, one must wonder if the moral, philosophical, and religious constraints against this course would progressively decrease with successive patients.

This consideration is the essence of the "wedge" or "slippery slope" argument, not only in relation to the individuals involved, but to society at large. Jean Rostrand bluntly describes the risk.

> A terrible precedent would be established if we agreed that a life could be allowed to end because it is not worth preserving.... After eliminating what was no longer human, the next step would be to eliminate what was not sufficiently human, and finally nothing would be spared except what fitted a certain ideal concept of humanity.[30]

In the view of Robert Veatch,

> Possibly tolerating active killing for mercy will lead to increase in other active killings, not because of any logical connection, but simply because those who are not careful may mistake one form of killing for another, or those who want to actively kill to benefit others will rationalize their actions by claiming that they are committed as acts of kindness to the recipient.[31]

Another argument against active euthanasia is that there is no absolute certainty in medicine (the reader is referred back to the paragraph on the "hopeless" patient on page 31). Active euthanasia of course ends any possibility of improvement in an irreversibly comatose patient, however remote or unprecedented such improvement may be. Even the best medical judgment is not entirely in-infallible.

An additional consideration is the patient-doctor relationship based on trust. Would this be eroded by instances of active euthanasia? There would likely be no problem when the patient and family knew the doctor well and the relationship was well established. Yet with the increasing specialization of the medical profession and the need to refer patients with complicated problems to doctors previously unknown to the patient and family, there might not be time for trust to build up before decisions were needed. It is unthinkable, however, that decisions for active euthanasia would be taken unilaterally, before thorough discussion with the family and without their agreement. Nevertheless, there is a great difference between the attitude of society to the individual doctor and to the corporate medical profession. While active euthanasia might not weaken individual patient-doctor relationships, it could engender a general distrust of the profession in society at large.

In ending this section, it should be made explicit that, if ever *active euthanasia* were to be legalized, the law should state unequivocally that no doctor could be compelled to act contrary to his or her beliefs and conscience.

Legal Considerations

The intentional termination of life to end suffering is a crime and may be either murder or manslaughter, whether death results from positive action or is the consequence of refraining from life-sustaining treatment. The Criminal Code of Canada defines homicide as follows: "A person commits homicide when, directly or indirectly, by any means, he causes the death of a human being (a) by means of an unlawful act, or (b) by criminal negligence" (Section 205). A death is defined as murder "where the person who causes the death of a human being, means to cause his death." (Section 212).

The Code also states that a person is guilty of criminal negligence when he, "in doing anything or in omitting to do anything that is his duty to do, shows wanton or reckless disregard for the lives or safety of other persons" (Section 202). When a patient (or the family on his behalf) entrusts his care to a doctor who accepts him, a contract is implied between the two, and therefore the doctor owes a legal duty of care to the patient. It is further stated that "everyone who undertakes to administer surgical or medical treatment to another person or to do any other act that may endanger the life of another person is, except in case of necessity, under a legal duty to have and to use, reasonable knowledge, skill and care in so doing" (Section 198). Moreover "where a person causes bodily injury to a human being that results in death, he causes the death of that human being notwithstanding that the effect of the bodily injury is only to accelerate his death from a disease or disorder arising from some other cause" (Section 209).

Relatives and doctors have been prosecuted for murder in Britain and the United States when positive action to achieve active euthanasia has been taken. Usually, however, they have been acquitted by sympathetic juries on the technical grounds of temporary insanity or because criminal intent has not been proven. Prosecutions for criminal negligence, when death is caused or accelerated by refraining from or withdrawing treatment, have not often been pressed, one reason being that the responsible person clearly has not shown a wanton and reckless disregard for life. The courts have refused either to prosecute or else to convict in those situations in which a doctor has refrained from treatment for humanitarian reasons, or when large doses of drugs, intended to relieve pain, have hastened or caused death.

As an example, the records indicate that in a period of nine years the College of Physicians and Surgeons of the Province of Quebec was asked to investigate only one incident of euthanasia. In that case the physician was charged by a member of the family with having violated medical ethics, but was eventually cleared of any blame.[32]

Do our present laws, legal processes and sanctions, concerning matters of life and death in a medical context, adequately protect the rights and interests of the individuals involved? It may be argued that our laws and legal doctrines have to a large extent remained fixed in the past, with no account being taken of the new gains and threats posed by advances in medical technology and the evolution of society's values. The law appears to provide little security or certainty to patients, doctors, or the courts on the issues of preserving, or not preserving under certain conditions, the lives of those who are terminally ill, irreversibly comatose, or seriously defective. Actual practice is often contrary to legal theory, and there is a considerable gap between traditional values articulated in law and the interpretation of changed values by judge and jury.[33]

If it is morally right to refrain from treatment or to give treatment which may secondarily hasten death in certain patients, it ought not to be a violation of the law. For this reason, some doctors would like the law changed to legalize and regulate the *de facto* discretionary situation. They would also like to be protected from the possibility of criminal prosecution, initiated for example by relatives who do not concur in the doctor's decision, even though the patient wishes it. Indeed, if a rational patient has requested that a certain treatment be discontinued or not initiated with the aim of not prolonging his life, or that another treatment be given with the aim of ending it, is it moral and should it be legal for the doctor to accede to this request? What bearing should the opinion of the family have on the moral or legal aspects of the joint decision of patient and doctor? Other doctors would prefer the present quasi-legal status to continue, arguing that to conform to the requirements of a new law would complicate, protract, and depersonalize decisions which now are made with concern and expedition by those intimately involved.

Some argue that legally to permit the termination of life to end severe, uncontrollable suffering, would lead to abuse and that the principle of respect for life would be jeopardized. While society expects doctors to relieve suffering, it also expects them to preserve life and restore health. Moreover, pressure might be put on patients, either by family, medical attendants, or society in general, for improper reasons, such as financial and economic or just for mere convenience, so that a request that his life be terminated might not represent the patient's real wishes. This pressure might be overt, covert, or merely imagined by the patient.

However, some lawyers hold that it is possible to frame a law that would prevent abuse and safely cover all situations in which life could be ended to relieve severe suffering in terminal illness. It would have to stipulate, as an absolute prerequisite, a request by the patient, when rational, or by the immediate family, when the patient is legally incompetent. The request would have to be reaffirmed over a period of days, in case one wished to change one's mind. Such a law, while protecting doctors, would also protect the helpless who could not protect themselves. In the case of the "incompetent" patient, a prior statement made by an adult while still rational, setting out the circumstances in which he wished to continue living and those in which he wished his life to be ended or not prolonged, would be given due weight.

A statement of this kind is called a "living will." In California it has been given legal status in the Natural Death Act of 1976. A simple printed form is voluntarily executed by a competent adult and duly witnessed. This permits the attending physician to withhold or withdraw life-sustaining treatment when the patient becomes terminally ill or is mortally injured. The act does not authorize any affirmative action to end life (active euthanasia), and it is applicable to a limited range of patients. This was done to satisfy the pro-life groups and certain church organizations who eventually agreed to the act. It is worth noting, however, that one of the main purposes of the act was to settle a variety of legal issues, especially problems arising from professional malpractice suits. A number of other states in the Union have since passed similar legislation.

A bill dealing with the same matter was introduced in the Ontario Legislature in 1977. It did not come to third reading because a provincial general election was called. Moreover, it had been argued that the bill was beyond the competence of a provincial legislature. Since the problem of malpractice suits has not so far occurred in Canada to the same degree as in the United States, it is questionable whether such legislation is needed in this country at this time. Although there is in Canada no legal sanction of a living will, any person can complete a statement* requesting that he be allowed to die and not be kept alive by artificial means or "heroic measures," should circumstances arise when there is no reasonable expectation that he will recover from physical or mental disability. Such a statement may carry moral weight or even obligation with those who care for the patient but does not confer legal protection on them.

Leaving Canadian law as it is at present allows life and death decisions to rest on the diverse values and ethics held by individual doctors and other health care personnel. Society may feel that this is a burden and a power which doctors should not be compelled or allowed to bear and exercise by themselves. Perhaps the medical and allied professions, the patient and the public deserve and require more ethically sensitive, uniformly applicable laws or guidelines than now exist. Some form of legislation other than criminal law, or possibly non-legislative action, might better attain this purpose.[34] One must ask if uniform application is possible in situations which are so variable, even unique.

One recoils from the implications of the Saikewicz decision by the Massachusetts Supreme Judicial Court in November 1977. Saikewicz was 67 years old and profoundly retarded. He was found to have a symptomless form of leukemia for which chemotherapy offered only a moderate chance of temporary remission. The treatment would be painful. Because he would not understand what was happening, he might have to be restrained. Legal permission to withhold treatment was sought and obtained. However, the written judgment ruled in effect that all questions about initiating,

---

*Obtainable from the Euthanasia Educational Council, 250 West 57th Street, New York, N.Y. 10019 U.S.A.

ending, or continuing life-preserving therapy for legally incompetent patients must be subject to judicial decision. The usual court delays would then be compounded by the judicial appointment of a legal guardian for the patient, to present arguments against the petition sought, in an adversary proceeding. In so deciding, the court displayed a total distrust of the current medical system to handle life and death decisions with any degree of equity and sensitivity.[35] Moreover, the court declined to formulate guidelines for emergency situations involving incompetent patients, stating that this "is better left to the *legislative branch.*" In other words, when emergencies require decisions which could not have prior judicial approval, doctors must not be allowed to use their professional judgment but most be guided by government regulations, previously laid down by legislation.[36]

We must, at all costs, avoid a similar situation in Canada. Decisions made in the current manner have not always been in the patient's best interest, but there is little reason to think that any other system so far conceived would be more workable or less liable to error.[37] Our aim should be to arrange the legal situation in such a way that decisions can be made by the doctor and the patient (or his family) with a proper regard for society's values, and yet with the least distress to the family, and minimal damage to the dignity and personal integrity of the patient.[38]

Who Should Decide and How?

"Life is short, the art long, the occasion instant, experiment perilous, decision difficult." These words, attributed to Hippocrates, sum up the situation that often confronts those caring for the dying. Should it be agreed that in some circumstances the best possible course is to relieve suffering by allowing life to end, then we are faced with the question of who should make the decision. In the case of the rational patient, it goes without saying that in ethics and under the law his or her wishes must be the prime determinant. We have seen that, at the present time, the decision for the incompetent patient is made in effect by the doctor, though concurred in by the relatives. Many believe that this is indeed the doctor's proper province. He is in the position to insure that proper medical consultation is obtained before declaring a patient's condition hopeless, that the relatives receive sympathetic and thorough explanation, and that they are exposed to broadly-based advice, including support from their pastor or the hospital chaplain. The doctor usually finds himself leading all those involved to a decision and is often responsible for consoling and comforting after the decision has been reached.[39] Not all doctors, however, are sufficiently motivated to accept fully this demanding role.

Others think that the decision should be made by the family with the counsel of their pastor or the chaplain, in conjunction with the doctor. The family must be fully informed of the consequences of consenting to or withholding treatment, and a period of time should be allowed between reaching a decision and its enactment. This opinion differs from the previous one only in its lesser emphasis on the role of the doctor and its view that the decision is not his exclusive province.

A third opinion advocates the formation of hospital committees, such as those in New Jersey. Termed *prognosis* rather than *ethics* committees in this state, these are not really concerned to decide ethical or legal matters but instead assist the doctors primarily involved in the determination of the patient's medical condition. The committees, which are composed of doctors not in the treating group and usually from outside the particular hospital, should be able to act quickly and equitably.[40] They provide safeguards both for patients and doctors, and they diffuse responsibility. Such committees might, under new legislation, assume a legal status and allow courses of action not now undertaken because of concern for legal liability. However, objections to committees are raised because they depersonalize decisions that should be made intimately, and indeed, it is difficult to convey to a committee all the variable elements of each individual case. A committee's decision tends to be less sensitive than that of the small group primarily involved.

Although one speaks easily of "informed consent," one must appreciate that this requires a certain level of educated intelligence which is not always present. Not infrequently there is not only the barrier of ignorance to cope with, but also of language and culture. Even when these problems are absent, the stress of the situation may impair the ability of the patient or of his family to understand what the doctor is saying and to think through the alternative courses of action. Their natural emotions make it exceptionally hard for them to be truly autonomous. The doctor must be prepared to spend a lot of time with the patient or his family and should seek the help of their pastor or the hospital chaplain. The patient or his relatives need accurate information about the diagnosis and prognosis and the probable outcome of alternative courses of care, all of this simply and sympathetically explained. Finally, the doctor must try to bring them to a decision, without pressure or bias.

Much of a doctor's difficulty in this situation arises because the values of the dying patient may be quite different from his own. This brings us to the all-important question: "On whose value system should the decision be based?"[41] It can confidently be stated that the values of the immediate family, of those who provide medical care, or of society and economics should not be the basis of decision. The chief consideration should be the values of the patient as he or she is able to enunciate them or, if unable, as the doctor and the immediate family are able by responsible discussion to understand them. Such an approach is consistent with the autonomy God has allowed us. We should also emphasize that it is the duty of Christians, in this field as in all others, to try to persuade society that the highest values are those proclaimed in the Christian gospel.

The Influence of Economics

We have just stated that the choice of life or death should not be made on the basis of economic considerations. We must therefore consider whether, in practice, the costs of medical treatment influence these decisions. One often hears the argument that continued treatment of the "hopeless" patient imposes an unfair burden on our society and may indeed deplete resources that are limited and needed by less seriously ill patients. In the case of a patient in irreversible coma, this argument would seem acceptable because the person in such a patient is already dead and only biological life remains.[42]

Generally speaking, however, we should surely assume that the developed, affluent countries of the western world can and should afford the costs of ordinary medical care for all their citizens. They have sophisticated health systems, and access to these, in most western countries, is not governed by personal finances but is open to all. If the cost of ordinary care in our society is a factor in making decisions about the seriously sick, then surely our priorities are in disorder and not in accord with theological principles. Society can have no right on economic grounds to demand the cessation of treatment because the life of a sick person does not appear to be meaningful or valuable. Earlier it was asserted that all persons have a unique value which is not measured by their contribution to society nor by how old or sick they may be. The moral claims of the individual person should take precedence over those of society. The patient's right to continued care, and to that which promotes his highest good, outweighs the right of society to be freed of a burden.[43]

The situation would appear to be different when it comes to "extraordinary" care. This is often exceptionally expensive and consumes an undue proportion of the medical budget. It frequently requires an excessive amount of time and effort by a large number of medical personnel for benefits which are limited to relatively few patients, with dubious prospects of success. An example of such extraordinary care is heart transplants; these indeed, as of 1980, are not approved by the medical profession at large because of generally poor results, quite apart from the cost. Much of this type of treatment is experimental, and though it must be pursued if medicine is to advance, it should be conducted in a few university institutions only and be financed by grants from charitable trusts and professional organizations, as well as by special government grants outside the regular medical budget. Our attitude to extraordinary care, in distinction to care that is ordinary, should properly be governed by a realistic stewardship of the resources available to us for medical treatment.

In the recent years of fiscal restraint, there has been stern and increasing restriction of governmental financing of medical care. This has compelled doctors to give thought to medical costs and has inevitably influenced considerations about continuing life-supporting treatment for some patients. Present financial limitations have reduced the number of hospital beds, restricted the hiring of nursing and other paramedical personnel, and sharply curtailed the purchase of new and additional medical equipment.

Doctors have been compelled by these circumstances to consider a cost benefit factor in their care both of classes of patients and of individual patients. It may be that a new medical program for a certain group of patients is thought to be desirable. The response of government often is that the monies needed must be found by reducing care in other areas rather than through the provision of additional funds. Sometimes a patient may not be transferred to an intensive care unit for lack of beds or nursing staff, or another patient may be transferred prematurely from this unit to a regular ward. The nursing coverage of regular wards, at least on evening and night shifts and at weekends, is often minimal and barely sufficient for patient supervision and treatment, especially if one of them is dying. Two patients may need the same vital medical equipment when only one apparatus is available. Nevertheless, the amount of expensive equipment that a hospital stocks — for example, infant incubators — must be related to the expected use of it. It is unreasonable to squander resources on stocking enough equipment to cope with exceptional demands when it will nearly always stand idle.

In these circumstances, doctors have to decide how and by whom hospital beds and medical equipment should be used. The comparative values of individual lives are inevitably taken into consideration. Doctors are very perturbed at being forced into the rationing of medical care. It is probable that, in the best of circumstances, there will be some occasions when decisions may have to include these considerations, but certainly the allocation of financial resources should be such as to minimize these situations. The conditions of ordinary civilian life should not be coloured by the necessities imposed during war or other major disasters when medical facilities are overwhelmed by mass casualties. Then indeed a system of "triage" is inevitable, and treatment is necessarily withheld from those whose injuries are so severe that recovery is doubtful and whose treatment would divert care from those who could benefit.

There is certainly a responsibility on the part of the authorities, and on the medical profession in particular, to explore methods of providing adequate care that are less expensive than those presently utilized. Consideration should be given to increasing the employment of nurse-practitioners as an alternative to the wasteful and unnecessary use of medical practitioners. Day hospitals and the performance of lesser operations without overnight admission (day surgery) should be expanded. Custodial care, in nursing homes and extended care facilities for incapacitated persons who do not require medical treatment, costs less than accommodation in acute care hospitals, and the patients can receive more appropriate and concerned attention from staff who are not involved with more acutely ill patients.

In these institutions the nursing and social components assume a relatively larger role. They are geared to look after patients who are predominantly geriatric, and all the staff should be trained and experienced in this specialized branch of health care. Much of the treatment needed by such patients is ongoing and does not require elaborate support facilities. This is in distinction to acute care institutions in which multiple, often expensive, diagnostic tests are needed, followed by the initiation of complex, though short term, treatment that is often surgical. There is need for more programs and facilities for long term care, not only for financial reasons but, more importantly, because the staff have the particular training and motivation to look after such patients. At the present time governments are reluctant to undertake the initial capital expenditures required, even though these programs promise subsequent economies in operation, quite apart from the benefits they can bring to patients. However, care must be taken to avoid merely adding more facilities onto an already overburdened institutional system.

Much greater emphasis should be placed on home care programs, including the extension of palliative care of the dying into the community. This requires adequate supportive systems of laundry, equipment, and visits by doctors and nurses.[44] Temporary institutional admissions should be available to provide a respite for those who care for patients at home. These arrangements are not only less expensive but more considerate of the needs and wishes of the patient and family. The study of Dr David Skelton, previously mentioned, has documented this forcefully.

> Of more than one hundred patients who were fully aware of the probable imminence of their own death, almost eighty percent expressed a deep desire to die in their own homes. For many this was the home in which they had lived and loved and coped with the problems that life had previously dealt to them. It should hardly be surprising to us that so many, therefore, would choose to remain there to die.
>
> Of the individuals studied, however, sixty-eight percent actually died in an institutional setting. This finding seems to be paralleled by that of other workers in the field. The majority of deaths in our modern society occur in institutions and away from the home — yet home is where most people would yearn to be. In this study there were several major reasons for the discrepancy between the actual and the desired place of death. In some cases it was an apparent unwillingness on the part of the health-care professionals to allow the patient to remain at home. In other instances there were apparent inadequacies of social supporting services. The lack of a simple night-sitter relief service or a subsidized laundry program may have led to

the inability of a family to continue caring at home. In most cases these necessary services were not highly sophisticated or costly, indeed many were those normally fulfilled, in "less advanced" eras, by friends of the family or neighbours. Severe symptomatic distress or serious nursing requirements were in some cases the reason for admission to hospital. Adequate home care and nursing services, together with the willingness of physicians to practice domicillary care, can even here, however, reduce the need for transfer to hospital. In a considerable number of instances, the patient himself appeared to have undergone a sudden change of mind and requested removal from his home. In such cases the change of mind was usually indicative of a new or unresolved problem. Such changes were as significant as those occurring in the vital signs, such as respiratory rate, pulse, or blood pressure. If time was taken to elicit the unspoken reason for the expressed change of mind, the basic issue could often be dealt with and relieved. It was highly significant to note that in at least ninety percent of these latter cases the difficulties arose out of communication breakdowns.[45]

It is argued that the expenditure of money, time, and effort required for extraordinary care would better be devoted to raising the level of care given to the bulk of the sick and injured. Moreover, it is surely true that there is no excuse in our affluent society for financial restrictions on ordinary medical care. It has been said that the moral worth of a society can be judged by the protection and care it gives to its weak and helpless members. To the extent that governments represent all of us, we each bear responsibility for the present constraints, and we ought to consider whether and how we should act to arrest and reverse the situation. This can be accomplished either by re allocation of monies in the total government budget or by higher taxation to increase the total available. Are we willing to accept higher taxes to eliminate considerations of cost in the ordinary care of seriously sick and dying patients? Is it morally important to reach medical decisions on the basis that every person has unique value that is not measurable in economic terms? If the answer to these questions is "yes," then we as individuals and the Church as a body are obligated to bring our concerns to the attention of government and of our individual elected representatives, and to press for a re-ordering of budget priorities.

3
The Christian Response to Death

The Realities of Death

Death and dying have become such a popular concern in recent years that we have been deluged with conferences, text books, lectures, films, television programs, and a steadily growing number of organizations endeavouring to relieve the difficulties facing the terminally ill, their next-of-kin, and others responsible for their care. At the same time it is deplorable that much contemporary literature has treated the subject in a sentimental and trivial way. Peter Steinfels describes the current trend.

> It is reflected in the titles of books like *Living Your Dying,* or *Death Is All Right,* or *To Die With Style!* Concluding an article comparing Ms Mannes's book to Stewart Alsop's *Stay of Execution,* a moving but unsentimental account of confronting death from cancer, Paul Ramsey warns that "the same outlook and program" which gave us "calisthentic sexuality," when "addressed to 'the last taboo' can only lead eventually and logically to the same thing: to 'calisthentic dying.'" How long before some *Joy of Dying* ("A Gourmet Guide to Passing Away") makes the best-seller lists?[1]

Because death involves separation from loved ones, we must not underestimate the grief that faces the dying patient. The passage from life to death has its own unique mystery. It is a new experience and can bring great apprehension. For some, the fear of death is the fear of the unknown. For others, the fear of death may arise from the progressive loss of autonomy and physical and mental capacity inherent in the dying process.

The dying patient will very naturally question his readiness to face this event. It is not uncommon for people at this time to receive a vision of their total life experience with all its unfinished business, its failings, and especially those words or actions that have offended others. Many terminal patients are plagued with questions such as: "Am I ready to face God?" "Will I survive the judgment?"

"Will He be angry with the things I have done in my life?" "Do I have enough faith?" When these questions predominate, death can give rise to real dread.

It is of the utmost importance that we recognize and deal with the realities facing the terminally ill. Certain experiences and questions are to be expected and must not be ignored or passed over lightly. At the same time we consider that there are other realities which can strengthen and support the person in his passage from life to death. We believe that through the resurrection of Christ, life triumphs over death. In this light we need no longer regard death with fear and anxiety. Moreover, for those who have already "died with Christ," eternal life can begin now, during bodily life, and come to fulfilment after death. When one believes firmly in this regeneration and its daily effect throughout life, the fear and tension of the unknown is lightened. In a very real sense it is not unknown because it is being experienced now.

It is also true that we live with the hope that our personhood will survive death and that in some way we will be able to recognize our loved ones and be recognized by them. Death will provide us with the opportunity to enrich our personal relationships and bring fulfilment to the whole of our life on earth, which can then be seen in its true perspective.

Reflecting on the significance of death, Bernard Häring suggests:

> For the Christian, death is neither a flight from the body into the rarefied air of "pure spirits" as suggested by much of the Hellenistic tradition nor an alienation from bodily reality. It is hope for the fullness of personal life, faith in the resurrection of the body and in the transfiguration of the whole person. It holds the promise of unity with the whole of creation, and therefore includes hope for a new heaven and a new earth, a transformation which goes beyond all experiences of present faith and love.[2]

Nevertheless, the prospects of God's judgment can weigh heavily on the minds of people facing death, and we need to respond to this. It would be contrary to one of the fundamentals of our Christian faith if we were to ignore our final assessment by God, but we would be committing a greater error if we did not reaffirm our belief in the mercy of God and the possibility of rebirth in Christ. The gospel is first and foremost a proclamation of the love of God and the joys he so eagerly wishes to bestow upon us.

It is our belief that these realities of the Christian life are the means of dealing with the realities of death, so that the passage from life to death may also be a passage to new life.

Preparing for Death

Much has been written about the process of dying and the various stages one may experience, such as denial, anger, depression, bargaining, and peaceful acceptance.[3] An understanding of this process, both by the dying patient and the next-of-kin, is an invaluable aid in preparation for death. It should not be necessary, however, to repeat what has already been well documented, in particular by Elisabeth Kübler-Ross. We suggest that people take the opportunity to acquaint themselves with this information before they have to face their own dying or the death of someone close to them.

It is equally important for us to consider how our understanding of the Christian faith may help us prepare for death. We have spoken of death as a moment of separation, of loss, of entering the unknown, of receiving the promise of a new existence. We have also pointed out that a new life can in part be experienced here and now. We would like to think that our belief in the resurrection enables us to prepare ourselves and to taste something of that life which exists beyond death.

It is unfortunate that most of us associate the resurrection with an historic event or a future hope. We think of the resurrection of Jesus either as an event in the past, or in terms of a promise to share this experience in the future. Even though both statements are profoundly true, H.A. Williams has reminded us that the resurrection experience can be a present event. He says, "The miracle of our being given life beyond the grave is no greater than the miracle of our continually being given life here."[4]

Every time we receive the gift of new life, we enter into that resurrection experience. There can be no denying the fact that both physically and spiritually our lives always have the potential for being regenerated. Our lives are constantly changing. We receive new insights, undertake new tasks, establish new relationships, develop new skills, and as we all hope, acquire day by day a new awareness of God's will for us and of his presence in our lives. These are all resurrection experiences because they are moments when we receive new life.

We have to remember that every resurrection involves a death of some kind. Death always precedes resurrection. Thinking of this in terms of our own personal growth, we might illustrate these "death" and "new life" experiences in this way: a child must die to crawling in order to live for walking; a person must die to particular relationships in one family in order to live for a new relationship in marriage; a person must die to another in bereavement in order to live for a new set of relationships with others; a person must die to one job in order to live for a new style of work; a person must die to work in order to live for retirement. These are the "little deaths" constituting the variety of changes we must experience in order that growth and new life may come into being. It would seem that, as we face these "little deaths" constructively in the midst of life, we become better prepared to face the death of our physical bodies and the new spiritual life promised to us. H.A. Williams says again, "If we are ready for life in the sense of being open to its power and possibilities, then we are also ready for death. If we are aware of resurrection in the present, then we shall not be over-concerned about resurrection in the future."[5]

It may be argued that some of these little deaths only constitute a temporary release from a particular function or state of life, and in that sense are quite different from physical death, which is complete release and can never be retracted. A child who dies to crawling in order to walk may, if he wishes, return to crawling if his first steps prove unsuccessful. Similarly a retiree may return to work if he finds his retirement adjustment too difficult. There is, however, no second chance with the death experience, and this makes the transition far more difficult to face. Even though this should be acknowledged, it is still true that, if people find these minor deaths too difficult, it will be even more traumatic for them to face physical death.

It is at this point that we must issue a warning which may be seen as a sad commentary on our society. We have been called an acquisitive society — and correctly! We acquire but are loath to relinquish. We accumulate a wealth of things, of experiences, of acquaintances, of life itself — all of which can overburden us unless we are capable of relinquishing the old as we acquire the new. There is constant need to reassess the life we are carrying with us and, if necessary, die to something in order to live for something else. It is our firm belief that those who can adapt themselves to the rhythm of death and resurrection in this life will find themselves better prepared to face that ultimate moment when physical death will be the prelude to new spiritual life.

Facing Pain and Suffering

In the opening section of this report we remarked that people are more afraid of the process of dying than of death itself. People want to die with some dignity and with as high a degree of consciousness as possible until the final moment of death. This is sometimes hard to achieve if severe pain is involved and large doses of analgesics are needed to relieve it. Pain is a basic concern of the medical profession, which seeks not only to preserve life but to relieve suffering. There is an old saying that the physician's task is to cure rarely, relieve often, and comfort always. Fortunately, cure and relief can be attained more often now than in former years. However, we must also recognize that the treatment of disease may itself cause suffering. Sometimes life can only be preserved temporarily and at incredible cost in human suffering. For example, some chemotherapeutic drugs, while very beneficial in the treatment of some cancer patients, may produce distressing reactions. Rather than cure, these drugs frequently offer limited prolongation of existence and only slight possibility of a better quality of life for the remaining days. For these potential benefits, the dying patient must realize that the price is sometimes high. As in the management of all disease, the physician has to weigh the risks of undesirable side effects of a proposed course of treatment against the benefits that may reasonably be anticipated. What quality of life can the patient hope to enjoy from these procedures? How much suffering should an individual be expected to endure? All too often the treatment eventually becomes worse than the disease. The prospects for meaning and purpose in life then seem insufficient to justify measures that are medically possible but humanly unbearable. The prolongation of life seems less important than the comfort of the time that remains. We must recognize that the desires of a patient and of his family may conflict at this stage. The patient may fear the dying process more than death, the family may fear death more than the dying.

There are, however, problems associated with pain other than physical discomfort. It is interesting to note that one of the most common statements we hear from patients who are experiencing considerable discomfort is "What have I done to deserve this?" The underlying assumption behind this statement is that suffering is associated with evil. It is even possible that this belief may be partially sustained by the story of the fall, when pain and suffering only came into existence as a result of man's disobedience. It is not uncommon for us to hear people explaining the existence of hardship and suffering as "something which God has sent to try us." It is most unfortunate that suffering has been so closely aligned with evil.

We must face the fact that suffering is an inevitable part of the reality of life. Struggle and hardship have been an essential ingredient in the whole evolutionary process of creation. Species which have failed to engage in the struggle for growth have also endangered their survival. The human species is also aware that suffering can be beneficial; indeed, we might all agree that certain hardships in life have done more for us than occasions when everything has been simple and easy.

Since suffering is a fact of nature, it cannot be considered as inherently good or bad. There are, however, degrees of it which are both degrading and dehumanizing. There are occasions when hardship and distress seem to provide no benefit to the patient and, indeed, may be destructive to his well-being and personality. We think any suffering that becomes destructive to the growth of the human personality should be considered evil, and every effort should be made to get rid of it.

We have spoken of the elimination of suffering as the duty of the medical profession. It is also the responsibility of the medical profession to respect the fact that the patient may, in certain respects, know his own body better than the doctor. The relief of pain should be the combined effort of both doctor and patient. It also needs to be recognized that the relief of distress and suffering involves far more than physical remedies. Distress can in many instances be aggravated by emotional and spiritual problems. This brings us to the point where we must consider the total care of the dying person.

Care of the Dying

Our primary responsibility is to provide the best possible care for a patient who is preparing for death. Surely this is what Francis Bacon had in mind when he wrote in 1623, "I esteem it the office of a physician not only to restore health but to mitigate pain and dolours and not only when such mitigation may conduce to recovery, but when it may serve to make a fair and easy passage."[6]

In our view "a fair and easy passage" is the best definition of society's role in relation to the dying patient, but it must be admitted that easing the transition from life to death is something for which medical personnel are poorly trained and in which, for a number of reasons, they often serve the patient less than well. This may be due in part to the lack of training in counselling techniques, the reluctance to become emotionally involved, or the problem of providing the required amount of time that a patient needs during this transition.

However, serious attempts are being made to remedy the situation. These endeavours are based on the premise that whatever time is left to the dying patient, it is imperative that he continue to live with dignity and personal well-being. This can be achieved by offering particular medical care and skills.

The patient should be given the assurance that his physician, the nursing staff, his family and friends will support, console, and care for him to the end, so that he does not feel abandoned, lonely, and desolate. He should be assured of relief from distressing symptoms, pain, nausea, and difficulty in breathing. Every opportunity and encouragement should be given to enable both patient and family to speak openly about their grief and any other matters that may cause feelings of guilt after the death. People with experience are now urging that children, who are often sensitive to what is going on around them, should not be deceived when someone in the family is dying, but should be told the truth gently and helped to play their part in the family's response to the crisis. This can be a time for deep reconciliation between members of the family and also an opportunity to achieve spiritual peace with God.

These basic principles of care, which cover the physical, mental, emotional, and spiritual needs of the terminally ill person, have in some instances received special examination and implementation. The service being offered at the Palliative Care Unit in St Boniface General Hospital is a case in point. This hospital has made provision for a ward in which the terminally ill patient can live and die with comfort and dignity. Patients are encouraged to spend most of their time at home, always knowing that if symptoms become intolerable, or if personal care becomes too demanding for the family, admission will be available without difficulty. Because the emphasis at home is on security in facing discomfort and disability, there is no restrictive policy in diagnosis (although the large majority are cancer patients). Similarly, there is no restriction on the range of treatment provided, including radiotherapy, chemotherapy, and rarely, surgery. The in-patient service emphasizes the relief of symptoms and the emotional support of the patient and the family undergoing loss. There is a highly diversified care-team including nursing, medicine, social work, pastoral care, rehabilitation, dietetics, pharmacy, activities, and home care. There is a more intensive volunteer program than in any other unit in the hospital. Weekly conferences are held to review the physical, social, and emotional needs of all patients. This assures every patient that his concerns are being heard and dealt with. He also becomes very conscious that he is being cared for as a person.

Because this is one of few similar services in Canada, the unit has received considerable attention from visitors and the media. Staff have been invited to participate in many educational in-service programs for health-service personnel on the care of the dying. Students from a variety of health-care professions have had personal experience on the service. Dr David Skelton indicates the reasons why this service is needed.

> Our hospitals, contrary to popular opinion, are not bastions of cure, the site of the unfailing triumph of science and skill over death and disease. As Elisabeth Kübler-Ross has so dramatically pointed out, people do indeed die in our hospitals. Some seventy-five percent of all patients resident in our acute hospitals will not be cured; at best they will receive symptomatic relief for their ills. Of the twenty-five percent of patients who are more fortunate, as many as one half will probably have self-limiting disorders and, given adequate time, will recover spontaneously. Thus it is only in a relatively small proportion of patients that medical science effectively reverses the advancing tide of a pathological process. An increasing percentage of hospital patients are not acutely ill, but have chronic and degenerative disorders that strictly speaking are incurable and eventually will end in death. Often, unfortunately, the health-care professionals' education still fosters the image of a curative agent and tends to undervalue the supportive aspect of his vocation.
>
> It is not surprising, therefore, that many workers in the field of health care regard death not only as a personal threat, reminding us of our own mortality, but also as a challenge to professional status, since death may be viewed as a failure. Studies of

> hospital care of the dying patient, conducted on an international basis, have shown consistently that less time is spent with such patients, and greater delay occurs in providing attention to these individuals, than is the case for persons with a better prognosis. Many dying people apparently feel rejected and isolated in the midst of busy general hospitals, and their associated fears and symptomatic discomforts go unrelieved.[7]

Dr Skelton goes on to describe the kind of treatment which is offered in the St Boniface unit.

> Symptomatic treatment, undertaken in the most active manner, is the backbone of good medical care in the management of the dying patient. Pain relief is feasible in approximately ninety percent of cases, and favourable modification of the physical distress may be achieved in all but one or two percent of instances. The use of anticipatory analgesics is to be recommended; the patient should never be allowed to experience severe unrelieved discomfort. By anticipation and administration of medications before pain is actually felt, the patient's confidence and trust is maintained. Pain thresholds are affected by many factors over and above the structural somatic changes. Anxiety, loneliness, unresolved questions, embarrassment, difficulty in changing positions in bed or chair, toileting, and many other factors may influence pain perception. Again, a comprehensive approach to symptomatic relief is essential to ensure maximal beneficial results in this area of patient care.
> Other symptomatic problems such as breathlessness, nausea, vomiting, diarrhea, and offensive discharges are commonly encountered in this clinical situation. Here again, however, the rapid advances achieved in medical science have widened and deepened our ability to assist our patients. Although the spiritual, emotional, and social dimensions have to be appreciated, fully understood, and utilized, high clinical competence is still a *sine qua non* of palliative care.[8]

The focus of such care is summed up in these words.

> Our responsibility is to listen and hear, to develop as clear and realistic a concept of the problems as possible, to manipulate the environment appropriately and constructively, and above all to encourage and allow the dying person to draw on his own inner resources and strengths in order to provide, as far as pos-

> sible, the solutions to his own problems. In this way, despite erosion of his physical capacities, the individual retains self-respect, dignity, and identity.[9]

There are other models of health care being offered to the terminally ill in Canada. In some instances, palliative-care teams function throughout the whole hospital. Other models are designed to provide auxiliary services for the terminally ill at home. All of these efforts to improve the service and awaken the concern of the community for the terminal patient deserve the highest praise and the support of both church and society.

The Responsibility of the Church

It is our belief that any person who undertakes the responsibility of preparing someone for impending death is, in fact, putting his theology of death and resurrection into practice. To us such a task is of greatest importance and merits top priority.

We believe very strongly that Christians can fulfil this responsibility in a unique way. A study done at the Palliative Care Unit of the Royal Victoria Hospital, Montreal illustrates the point. It was discovered that the general level of stress experienced by this group of staff was noticeably higher than for staff in two other units in the hospital. The stress level decreased when certain staff members resigned. Dr David Shepherd made this assessment.

> Among staff who did not resign two factors seemed important: the meaning of religion to them (no one who stated that religion was very important resigned) and a venturesome and spontaneous personality. These factors are compatible with the nature of palliative care work, which is unique and innovative and calls for an unusual degree of dedication and commitment demanding thereby acceptance of personal risk in giving of oneself to others.[10]

We think the Church has a clear calling to undertake this work. We believe that both clergy and laity can be specially equipped for it and that every effort should be made to make them aware of their responsibility. There is a great need at the present time for church people to receive special training for the care of the terminally ill. Far too often there is a tendency to avoid such care. This arises not out of callousness but rather through feelings of inadequacy and helplessness. It is important, therefore, that clergy and laity receive training which will enable them to identify their own feelings about death and to develop the attitudes needed for the total care of the terminally ill.

We would see trust, openness, honesty, creativity, empathy, and a willingness to respect the individuality of the person concerned as fundamental. As we approach the dying person it would seem necessary that we recognize both our own mortality and the patient's life expectancy. Our attitude should not imply, "You are dying but I am living," but rather, "Your life, like mine, is fragile." In this way we resist the temptation to stigmatize such people, and we open ourselves to a genuine dialogue which can enrich both us and the dying person. We thereby come to recognize our own personhood, and this is one of the most important resources we have to enable others to be persons to the end.

Above all, the clergy and concerned lay people should take on the role of enablers. They can only do this if they are good listeners. They should try to help dying persons to become less dependent on their surroundings and those caring for them, and so to maintain as much autonomy as possible at this time. Dying patients need to become comfortable within themselves, and we can help by respecting their ability to be partially responsible for their own care. When all responsibility is assumed by others, the patient is deprived of the freedom and decision making that are fundamental to being a person. At all times we need to preserve those qualities of living which have always given meaning to personhood. In this way the Church affirms and fulfils to the end our Lord's mission: "I have come that men may have life, and may have it in all its fulness" (John 10:10. NEB). If Christians have a responsibility to the terminally ill, it is to be preoccupied with the sick person's life, not his death.

Both clergy and laity should also recognize their responsibility to act as advocates of the terminally ill. It is all too apparent that health-care services operate in certain ways that either ignore or underestimate the concerns of the terminally ill. Far too often the health professionals do not spend sufficient time with the patient to hear his concerns. There are two factors involved here. In many instances they are too busy to provide the patient with the time needed, and the patient, on his part, is fearful of bothering them. There are times when the patient remembers something later but is hesitant to voice his concerns. There are few people to whom the patient can turn without fear of upsetting the system. It is vital to find people who can establish a relationship of trust with the dying person and so "represent" the patient to other members of the health-care team. This could be seen as a position of advocacy, one which would benefit both patient and the caring community, and which Church people could readily fill.

We would urge that the terminally ill be given the maximum opportunity to spend their remaining time at home. This is contrary to the existing pattern where over 70 percent of Canadians die in institutions, often after a prolonged period of care. One of the reasons for such a pattern is the absence of adequate home care programs. It is also quite evident that we cannot at present expect major increases in government support in order to establish such programs. It is clear that an improvement in the care of the terminally ill will have to depend more and more on a reallocation of resources and on the work of volunteers. This has indeed become manifest in all the palliative care services in hospitals today. They find it impossible to function adequately without the additional support of volunteers.

The challenge to respond could not be put to a more relevant body than the Church. We are a people who have been commissioned by God to offer our services in a volunteer capacity. There is no other organization in the world which can claim as much experience and expertise in this role. It only remains for us to prepare ourselves to fulfil this responsibility and to do so with joy and gratitude that we have a special ministry in the service of our fellowman.

It is with a certain faith and a sure hope that we encourage the Church to recognize all these responsibilities and to fulfil them to the glory of God and the well-being of humanity.

Recommendations

A That the Church take every possible opportunity to influence those involved in care of the dying by providing active and continuing moral and spiritual guidance.

B *Education*

1 That the Church recognize its responsibility to provide educational programmes to foster a better understanding of the needs of the dying patient, of those responsible for the patient's welfare, and of the next of kin. These programs should focus on a number of specific areas.

a The elaboration, in the continuing education of clergy, of their special role with the dying patient and with their immediate families.

b The inclusion of similar training and experience within the academic and pastoral programs of theological colleges.

c Equipping the laity for effective ministry to the terminally ill in conjunction with the medical team and for service in volunteer home care programs of hospitals.

d The development in the Church and in society at large of a more realistic and wholesome attitude to and acceptance of the dying process and of death itself.

2 a That the Church urge local professional associations to initiate programs of continuing education for doctors and nurses to develop more skillful and compassionate care of the dying and bereaved.

b That the Church emphasize the importance of similar training in the curricula of all health care teaching institutions.

C *Patient Care*

1 That the Church actively support and encourage all persons and institutions which provide effective care for the terminally ill, such as the Palliative Care Units at the Royal Victoria Hospital, Montreal and at St Boniface Hospital, Winnipeg, and all those working toward the establishment of similar units in other hospitals.

2 That the Church make continuing representations to provincial governments for the provision of a growing scale of *small*, independent units for the care of terminal patients in which conditions allow the development of close relations between patients, their families, and those who care for them.
3 That the Church urge hospitals to expand home care programs in the community with the support of visiting nurses, physician home visits, and ancillary services so that dying patients may have the option of remaining at home in the care of their families.
4 That the Church initiate feasability studies for improving further the care of dying patients, in cooperation at the local level with appropriate medical boards, regional health councils, professional societies, provincial associations and other agencies, and that the findings be forwarded to provincial and federal governments.

D That these recommendations be carried out by widespread distribution of the report throughout the Anglican Church of Canada for study and discussion at the diocesan and parish levels and by action on an ecumenical basis at the national or local level, as most appropriate.

Summary

We believe that, if these recommendations are accepted and acted on widely, many of the ethical, social, medical and legal dilemmas that surround dying today, would be greatly alleviated.

Notes

Preface

1 Anglican Consultative Council — 3rd Report (Trinidad, 1976), pp. 30–2.

1 The Problem and Man's Response

1 Balfour M. Mount, "The problem of caring for the dying in a general hospital: the palliative care unit as a possible solution," *Canadian Medical Association Journal* 815 (2), (July 1976), pp. 119–21.

2 Donald Coggan, "On dying and dying well," *Crucible* (January -March 1977), p. 10 and *Proceedings of the Royal Society of Medicine* 70 (London, February 1977), p. 75.

3 Hugh Trowell, *The Unfinished Debate on Euthanasia* (London: SCM Press, 1973), p. 29. A case reported by W.St.C. Symmers in the *British Medical Journal* 1 (1968), p. 442.

4 Robert and Peggy Stinson, "On the Death of a Baby," *Atlantic Monthly* 244 (1) (July 1979), pp. 64–65.

5 M. Martin Halley and William F. Harvey, "Medical vs Legal Definitions of Death," *Journal of the American Medical Association* 204 (6), (May 1968), pp. 423–25.

6 Daniel C. Maguire, *Death by Choice* (New York: Doubleday, 1974), p. 17.

7 Report of the Ad Hoc Committee of the Harvard Medical School to Examine the Definition of Brain Death, "A definition of irreversible coma," *The Journal of the American Medical Association* 205 (6), (August 1968), pp. 337–40.

8 *Proceedings of the 107th Annual Meeting of the General Council of the Canadian Medical Association*, Toronto, 24–26 June 1974, Items 75–77, pp. 82–83.

9 Ian McColl Kennedy, "The Kansas statute on death — an appraisal" and Don Harper Mills, "The Kansas death statute: bold and innovative," *The New England Journal of Medicine* 285 (October 1971), pp. 946–50, pp. 968–69. See also a report by the Task Force on Death and Dying of the Institute of Society, Ethics, and the Life Sciences, "Refinements in criteria for the determination of death: an

appraisal" *The Journal of the American Medical Association* 221 (1), (July 1972), pp. 48–53; Roger B. Dworkin, "Death in context," and Alexander Morgan Capron, "The purpose of death: a reply to Professor Dworkin," *Indiana Law Journal* 48 (Summer 1973), pp. 623–46; Hans Jonas, "Against the stream: comments on the definition and redefinition of death," *Philosophical Essays: From Ancient Creed to Technological Man.* (Englewood Cliffs, N.J.: Prentice-Hall, 1974), pp. 132–40.

10 Law Reform Commission of Canada, *Criteria for the Determination of Death*, Working Paper 23 (Ottawa, 1979), pp. 58–59.

11 Robert M. Veatch, "Brain Death: Welcome Definition... or Dangerous Judgment?" *Hastings Center Report* 2 (5), (November 1972), p. 10.

12 Bernard Häring, *Medical Ethics*, (Notre Dame, Indiana: Fides Publishers 1973), pp. 132–33.

13 Joseph Fletcher, "Indicators of humanhood: a tentative profile of man," *Hastings Center Report* 2 (5), (November 1972), pp. 1–4.

14 R.B. Salter, "Modern medicine, genetics, and the future of mankind," *Annals of the Royal College of Physicians and Surgeons of Canada* 11 (3), (July 1978), pp. 209–17.

15 G.R. Dunstan, *The Artifice of Ethics* (London: SCM Press, 1974), p. 70.

16 Richard A. McCormick, "To Save or Let Die," *Journal of the American Medical Association* 229 (2) (1974), p. 175.

17 Edward W. Keyserlingk, *Sanctity of Life or Quality of Life in the context of ethics, medicine and law*, Law Reform Commission of Canada (Ottawa, 1979), p. 4.

18 Ibid., p. 42.

19 Ibid., p. 76.

20 Karl Barth, *Church Dogmatics* 3, "The Doctrine of Creation" 4, (Edinburgh: T&T Clark, 1961), p. 338–40.

21 Paul Ramsey, "The Morality of Abortion," in James Rachels, ed., *Moral Problems: A Collection of Philosophical Essays* (New York: Harper and Row, 1971), p. 45.

22 Bernard Häring, *Medical Ethics*, pp. 11–14.

23 Keyserlingk, *Sanctity of Life*, p. 60.

24 David Skelton, "A Testimony," *Dying: Considerations Concerning the Passage from Life to Death*, mimeographed draft (Anglican Church of Canada Archives, July 1979), pp. 58–59.

2 Decisions about Life and Death

1 R.S. Duff and A.G.M. Campbell, "Moral and Ethical Dilemmas in the Special Care Nursery," *New England Journal of Medicine* 289 (1973), p. 890.

2 Thomas O'Donnell, *Morals in Medicine* (Westminster, Md.: Newman Press, 1957), p. 66.

3 Report of the Clinical Care Committee of the Massachusetts General Hospital, "Optimum Care for Hopelessly Ill Patients," *New England Journal of Medicine* 295 (1976), p. 362.

4 Duff and Campbell, "Dilemmas," p. 890.

5 Karl Barth, *Church Dogmatics.* 3 "The Doctrine of Creation," 4 (Edinburgh: T & T Clark, 1961), p. 427.

6 R.H. Williams, "Our Role in the Generation, Modification and Termination of Life," *Archives of Internal Medicine* 124 (1969), p. 215; N.K. Brown et al, "The Preservation of Life," *Journal of the American Medical Association* 211 (1970), p. 76 and A. Shaw, J.G. Randolph, and B. Manard, "Ethical Issues in Pediatric Surgery: a national survey of Pediatricians and Pediatric Surgeons," *Pediatrics* 60 (1977), p. 588.

7 Statement by the American Medical Association House of Delegates, "The Physician and the Dying Patient," *Journal of the American Medical Association* 227 (1974), p. 728.

8 James Rachels, "Active and Passive Euthanasia," *New England Journal of Medicine* 292 (1975), p. 78.

9 Paul Ramsey, *The Patient as Person* (New Haven: Yale University Press, 1970), p. 151.

10 Hans Jonas, "The right to die," *Hastings Center Report* 8 (August 1978), p. 34.

11 E.J. Cassell, "The Function of Medicine," *Hastings Center Report* 7 (6), (December 1977), p. 16.

12 Cicely Saunders, "The Moment of Truth: Care of the Dying Person" in Francis G. Scott and Ruth M. Brewer, eds. *Confrontations of Death* (Oregon Centre for Gerontology, Corvallis, Oregon 1971), p. 119.

13 Pope Pius XII, "The Prolongation of Life," *The Pope Speaks* 4 (4), (1958), pp. 393–98.

14 Donald Coggan, "On Dying and Dying Well" *Crucible* (January–March 1977), p. 10. and *Proceedings of the Royal Society of Medicine* 70 (London, 1977), p. 75.

15 R.A. McCormick, "To Save or Let Die," *Journal of the American Medical Association* 229 (1974), p. 172.

16 Lamer, Mr. Justice Antonio. Speech to the 28th General Synod, Anglican Church of Canada, 15 August 1977, mimeographed (Anglican Church of Canada Archives).

17 Pope Pius XII, "The Prolongation of Life," pp. 393–98.

18 Report of the Ad Hoc Committee of the Harvard Medical School to Examine the Definition of Brain Death. "A Defini-tion of Irreversible Coma, "*Journal of the American Medical Association* 205 (1968), p. 337. See also, Conference of Medical Royal Colleges and their Faculties (UK), "Diagnosis of Death," *British Medical Journal* 2 (1976), p. 1187 and 1 (1979), p. 332. *Lancet* 2 (1976), p. 1069 and 1 (1979), p. 261; and "The Canadian Medical Association Statement on Death," *Canadian Medical Association Journal* 99 (1968), p. 1266.

19 Lamer, Speech.

20 D.P. Girvan, and C.A. Stephens, "Congenital Intrinsic Duodenal Obstruction: A twenty-year Review of its Surgical Management and Consequences," *Journal of Pediatric Surgery* 9 (1974), p. 833.

21 Lamer, Speech.

22 G.M. Hunt, "Implications of the Treatment of Myelomeningocoele for the Child and his Family," *Lancet* 2 (1973), p. 1308.

23 J. Lorber, "Early Results of Selective Treatment of Spina Bifida Cystica," *British Medical Journal* 4 (1973), p. 201.

24 G. Hunt et al. "Predictive Factors in Open Myelomeningocoele with Special Reference to Sensory Level," *British Medical Journal* 4 (1973), p. 197.

25 G.K. Smith, and E.D. Smith, "Selection for Treatment in Spina Bifida Cystica," *British Medical Journal* 4 (1973), p. 189.

26 M.D. Ames, and L. Schut, "Results of Treatment of 171 Consecutive Myelomeningocoeles — 1963 to 1968." *Pediatrics* 50 (1972), p. 466.

27 Duff and Campbell, *"Dilemmas,"* p. 890.

28 Eugene Fairweather, "The Child as Neighbour" *The Right to Birth,* (Toronto: Anglican Book Centre, 1976), p. 46.

29 Duff and Campbell, "*Dilemmas,*" p. 890.

30 John Rostrand in Edward W. Keyserlingk, *Sanctity of Life* or *Quality of Life,* Law Reform Commission of Canada (Ottawa, 1979), p. 22.

31 Robert Veatch, "Death, Dying and the Biological Revolution." (New Haven: Yale University Press, 1976), p. 89.

32 C.A. Gravenor, "Euthanasia: No Call for Heroics," *Canadian Doctor* (April 1976), p. 39.

33 Lamer, Speech.

34 *Ibid.*

35 W.J. Curran, Law-Medicine Notes "The Saikewicz Decision," *New England Journal of Medicine* 298 (1978), p. 499.

36 A.S. Relman, "The Saikewicz Decision; Judges as Physicians," *New England Journal of Medicine* 298 (1978), p. 508.

37 *Ibid.*

38 R.S. Morison, Memorandum "On Principle" to Dr David T. Roy, Centre for Bioethics, Montreal, 27 February 1978, p. 3.

39 F.J. Ingelfinger, "Bedside Ethics for the Hopeless Case," Editorial, *New England Journal of Medicine* 289 (1973), p. 914.

40 Curran, "Saikewicz Decision," p. 499.

41 S.H. Imbus, and B.E. Zawacki, "Autonomy for Burned Patients when Survival is Unprecedented," *New England Journal of Medicine* 297 (1977), p. 308.

42 Lamer, Speech.

43 *Ibid.*

44 S. Malkin, "Care of the Terminally Ill at Home," *Canadian Medical Association Journal* 115 (1976), p. 129.

45 David Skelton, "A Testimony," "*Dying: Considerations Concerning the Passage from Life to Death,* mimeographed draft (Anglican Church of Canada Archives, July 1979), pp. 60–61.

3 The Christian Response to Death

1 Peter Steinfels and Robert M. Veatch, eds., *Death Inside Out* (New York: Harper & Row, 1975), p. 3.

2 Bernard Häring, *Medical Ethics* (Notre Dame, Indiana: Fides Publishers, 1973), p. 124.

3 Elisabeth Kübler-Ross, *On Death and Dying* (New York: The Macmillan Company, 1970).

4 H.A. Williams, *True Resurrection* (New York: Harper & Row, 1974), p. 177.

5 *Ibid.*, p. 180.

6 Francis Bacon, *Philosophical Works,* trans. by Ellis and Spedding and ed. by J.M. Robertson (Freeport, N.Y.: Books for Libraries, 1970), p. 106.

7 David Skelton, "A Testimony," *Dying: Considerations Concerning the Passage from Life to Death,* mimeographed draft (Anglican Church of Canada Archives, July 1979), p. 57–58.

8 *Ibid.*, pp. 62–63.

9 *Ibid.*, p. 59.

10 David A.E. Shepherd, "Principles and practices of palliative care," *Canadian Medical Association Journal* 116 (March 1977), p. 526.

Selected Bibliography

Books

Decisions About Life and Death, A Problem in Modern Medicine. London: The Church Assembly Board for Social Responsibility, Church Information Office, Church House, Dean's Yard, London, England, 1965.

On Dying Well, An Anglican Contribution to the Debate on Euthanasia. London: Church Information Office, 1975. Official documents produced by the Church of England. The earlier represents a great deal more research. In England there has been considerable debate on the introduction of a Voluntary Euthanasia Bill; hence there is emphasis in the documents on the feasibility of such a bill.

Alsop, Stewart. *Stay of Execution: A Sort of Memoir.* New York: J.P. Lippincott, 1973. A personal account of the author's experience and thoughts about death as he endured his struggle with cancer, finally fatal.

Ashley, B.M. and O'Rourke, K.D. *Health Care Ethics: A Theological Analysis.* St. Louis, Miss.: The Catholic Hospital Association, 1978.

Behnke, J.A. and Bok, Sissela, eds. *The Dilemmas of Euthanasia.* Garden City: Doubleday, Anchor Books, 1975. Includes articles on euthanasia and the care of the dying, legal aspects of euthanasia and physicians' attitudes towards the treatment of critically ill patients.

Callahan, Daniel. *The Tyranny of Survival and Other Pathologies of Civilized Life.* New York: Macmillan, 1973.

Campbell, A.V. *Moral Dilemmas in Medicine.* Baltimore: Williams and Wilkins, 1972. This short text includes clear explanations and comparisons of such fundamentals as the principle of double effect, "extraordinary means," Kant's categorical imperative, act and rule utilitarianism, psychological theories of morality and the principle of "reverence for life."

Cutler, D.R., ed. *Updating Life and Death.* Boston: Beacon Press, 1968. Paperback edition, 1969. Essays by well-known ethicists. Three deal with death and dying and one with the sanctity of life.

Downing, A.B., ed. *Euthanasia and the Right to Death; the Case for Voluntary Euthanasia.* London: Peter Owen, 1969. Contains a number of essays, advocating and criticizing the case for voluntary euthanasia.

Dunstan, G.R. *The Artifice of Ethics.* London: S.C.M. Press, 1974.

Fletcher, Joseph. *Morals and Medicine.* Princeton University Press, 1954. Paperback edition, Boston: Beacon Press, 1960. Medical ethics concerning euthanasia are analyzed. Emphasis is on the patient's right to know the truth about his condition and sections on keeping the patient alive and on moral responsibility are included.

Garfield, C.A. *Psychosocial Care of the Dying Patient.* New York: McGraw-Hill, 1978.

Gunther, John. *Death Be Not Proud.* New York: Harper and Row, 1971. A memoir to his seventeen year old son, who died after a series of operations for brain tumour.

Häring, Bernard. *Medical Ethics.* Notre Dame, Indiana: Fides Publishers, 1973.

Hendin, David. *Death as a Fact of Life.* New York: W.W. Norton, 1973. New thinking about legal, medical and psychological aspects of death by a medical journalist. It is written for the general public.

Hinton, J.M. *Dying.* Baltimore: Penguin Books, 1967. The rational and irrational emotions associated with death are discussed by a psychiatrist who has long been concerned with patients suffering from incurable illness. Chapters include fear of death and dying, physical distress in the terminal illness, speaking of death with the dying, prolonging life and hastening death and reactions to bereavement.

Jackson, E.N. *You and Your Grief.* New York: Channel Press, 1964. A brief statement by a minister to the mourner on dealing with his own grief and that of his children.

Keyserlingk, E.W. *Sanctity of Life or Quality of Life in the context of ethics, medicine and law.* Law Reform Commission of Canada, Ottawa, 1979.

Kluge, E.W. *The Practice of Death.* New Haven: Yale University Press, 1975.

Kohl, Marvin. *The Morality of Killing: Sanctity of Life, Abortion and Euthanasia.* New York: Humanities Press, 1974.

Kohl, Marvin, ed. *Beneficent Euthanasia.* Buffalo: Prometheus Books, 1975. Argues the case for euthanasia, both passive and active (assisting the death of a massively injured or terminally ill patient). At the same time, the dangers accompanying euthanasia and the special problems it presents for physicians and families are discussed.

Kubler-Ross, Elisabeth. *On Death and Dying.* New York: Macmillan, 1969. A concrete and practical discussion of what the dying have to teach the living. Contains a description of the stages through which the dying generally pass and which can usefully be considered as stages of the grief process.

Kubler-Ross, Elisabeth, ed. *Death: the Final Stage of Growth.* Englewood Cliffs, N.J.: Prentice Hall, 1975. A collection of articles, letters and poems.

Labby, D.H., ed. *Life or Death: Ethics and Options.* Seattle: University of Washington Press, 1968.

Ladd, John, ed. *Ethical Issues Relating to Life and Death.* New York: Oxford University Press, 1979.

LeShan, Lawrence. *You Can Fight for Your Life.* New York: N. Evans, A Jove Book, 1978.

Lewis, C.S. *A Grief Observed.* London: Faber and Faber, 1961. A response to the death of his wife. He concludes that bereavement is an integral part of the experience of love.

Maguire, D.C. *Death by Choice.* New York: Doubleday, 1974. Presents discussions on various attitudes towards death along with general concepts surrounding euthanasia.

Oden, T.C. *Should Treatment be Terminated? Moral Guidelines for Christian Families and Pastors.* New York: Harper and Row, 1976.

Rachels, James, ed. *Moral Problems: a Collection of Philosophical Essays.* New York: Harper and Row, 1971.

Ramsey, Paul. *The Patient as Person.* New Haven: Yale University Press, 1970. The Lyman Beecher lectures at Yale University. A Christian ethicist deals with such topics as experimentation and consent, definitions of death, care for the dying, transplantation and scarce medical resources.

Ramsey, Paul. *Ethics at the Edges of Life.* New Haven: Yale University Press, 1978. The Bampton Lectures in America.

Solzhenitsin, A. *Cancer Ward.* New York: Bantam Books, 1969.

Steinfels, Peter and Veatch, R.M., eds. *Death Inside Out.* New York: Harper and Row, 1975. A group of noted doctors, ethicists, social scientists and critics discuss such issues as the shifts in attitudes towards death over the past eight centuries, patterns of death in modern institutions, the 'death with dignity' controversy and the changing relationship of medicine and the dying.

St. John-Stevas, Norman. *Life, Death and the Law.* Cleveland: World Publishing, Meridian Books, 1961.

Tolstoy, Leo. *The Death of Ivan Illyich.* New York: Signet Books, New American Library, 1960.

Trowell, Hugh. *The Unfinished Debate on Euthanasia.* London: S.C.M. Press, 1973. A good resume of the debate on euthanasia. Contains three important appendices: "The Problem of Euthanasia," a report of the

Special Panel appointed by the Board of Science and Education, British Medical Association; "Doctors and Euthanasia," a rejoinder to the previous appendix by the Voluntary Euthanasia Society; and an analysis of the Voluntary Euthanasia Bill (1969).

Vaux, Kenneth, ed. *Who shall Live? Medicine, Technology, Ethics.* Philadelphia: Fortress Press, 1970. A report of the Houston Conference on Ethics in Medicine and Technology, 1968.

Veatch, R.M. *Death, Dying and the Biological Revolution.* New Haven: Yale University Press, 1976. The major issues in this book are the definition of death, the prolongation of life versus euthanasia, the patient's right to obtain information on his condition and to refuse treatment and the transplantation of organs from the newly dead.

Weber, L.J. *Who shall Live? The Dilemma of Severely Handicapped Children and its Meaning for Other Moral Questions.* Toronto: Paulist Press, 1976.

Williams, Glanville. *The Sanctity of Life and the Criminal Law.* New York: Knopf, 1957. Makes a comparison of the legal implications involved in suicide and euthanasia. Discusses euthanasia in religious, criminal and legal lights.

Williams, H.A. *True Resurrection.* New York: Harper and Row, 1974.

Periodicals

Bibliography of Society, Ethics and the Life Sciences. Published and updated annually by The Hastings Center, Hastings-on-Hudson, N.Y.

Admundsen, D.W. "The Physician's Obligation to Prolong Life." *Hastings Center Report* 8, (August 1978). pp. 23–30.

Alvarez, W.C. "Care of the Dying." *Journal of the American Medical Association,* 150 (2), (1952). pp. 86–91.

Annas, George. "The Incompetent's Right to Die; the Case of Joseph Saikewich." *Hastings Center Report* 8 (1) (1978). pp. 21–23.

Ayd, F.J. "The Hopeless Case." *Journal of the American Medical Association.* 181 (13), (1962). pp. 1099–1102.

Baylor Law Review (Winter 1975). Symposium on Euthanasia.

Beecher, H.K. "After the 'definition of irreversible coma'." *New England Journal of Medicine* 281 (1969). pp. 1070–1.

Bok, Sissela. "Personal Directions for Care at the End of Life." *New England Journal of Medicine* 295 (1976). p. 367.

Bok, Sissela and Ramsey, Paul. "The Leading Edge of the Wedge." *Hastings Center Report* 1 (December 1971). p. 9.

Capron, A.M. and Kass, L.R. "A Statutory Definition of the Standards for Determining Human Death: an Appraisal and a Proposal." *University of Pennsylvania Law Review* 121 (1972). pp. 87–118.

Clouser, K.D.: "The Sanctity of Life: an Analysis of a Concept." *Annals of Internal Medicine* 78 (1973). p. 119. He shows that the important elements of this concept are already subsumed under other and more defensible rules of ethics.

Fletcher, George. "Prolonging Life: some Legal Considerations." *Washington Law Review* 42 (1967). pp. 999–1016.

Fletcher, John. "Attitudes towards Defective Newborns." *Hastings Center Studies* 2 (January 1974). p. 21.

Fletcher, Joseph. "Four Indications of Humanhood — the Enquiry Matures." *Hastings Center Report* 4 (6) (December 1974). pp. 4–7.

Fox, J.E. "Reflections on Cancer Nursing." *American Journal of Nursing* 66 (1966). p. 1317.

Fried, Charles. "Terminating Life Support: Out of the Closet." *New England Journal of Medicine* 295 (1976). p. 390.

Garland, Michael. "Politics, Legislation and Natural Death: the Right to Die in California." *Hastings Center Report* 6 (October 1976). pp. 5–6.

Jonas, Hans. "The Right to Die." *Hastings Center Report* 8 (August 1978). pp. 31–36.

Jonsen, A.R. et al. "Critical Issues in New-Born Intensive Care: a Conference and Policy Proposal." *Pediatrics* 55 (1975). pp. 756–68.

Jonsen, A.R. and Lister, George. "New-born Intensive Care: the Ethical Problems." *Hastings Center Report* 8 (1) (February 1978), p. 15.

McCormick, R. "The Quality of Life, the Sanctity of Life." *Hastings Center Report* 8 (1) (February 1978), pp. 30–36.

Mount, B.M. "Palliative Care of the Terminally Ill." *Annals of the Royal College of Physicians and Surgeons of Canada* 11 (1978). p. 202.

Rabkin, M.T. et al. "Orders not to Resuscitate." *New England Journal of Medicine* 295 (1976). p. 364.

Ramsey, Paul. "Death's Pedagogy." *Commonweal* 100 (September 1974). pp. 497–502.

Ramsey, Paul. "Prolonged Dying: Not Medically Indicated." *Hastings Center Report* 6 (1) (February 1976). pp. 14–17.

Ramsey, Paul. "The Saikewicz Precedent: What's Good for an Incompetent Patient?" *Hastings Center Report* 8 (6) (December 1978). pp. 36–42.

Reid, Robert. "Spina Bifida: the Fate of the Untreated." *Hastings Center Report* 7 (4) (August 1977). p. 16.

Robertson, J.A. "Involuntary Euthanasia of Defective New-Borns: a Legal Analysis." *Stanford Law Review* 27 (1975). pp. 213–269.

Robitscher, Jonas. "The Right to Die." *Hastings Center Report* 2 (September 1972). p. 11.

Saunders, Cicely. "Care of the Dying." *Nursing Times* 72 (1976). pp. 1003, 1049, 1089, 1133, 1203, and 1247.

Shaw, Anthony: "Defining the Quality of Life." *Hastings Center Report* 7 (5) (October 1977). p. 11.

Toch, R. et al. "Management of the Child with a Fatal Disease." *Clinical Pediatrics* 3 (1964). pp. 418–427.

Veatch, Robert: "Death and Dying: the Legislative Options." *Hastings Center Report* 7 (5) (October 1977). pp. 5–8.

"Who Should Decide? The Case of Karen Quinlan." *Christianity and Crisis* 35 (1976), pp. 322–31.

Audio-Visual Aids

Many of the listed aids are available locally from public libraries, provincial Departments of Health, university and college libraries, and from church organizations. For films, consult also the yellow pages of the telephone directory under the heading Motion Picture Film Libraries and (for commercial outlets) under Motion Picture Film Distributors.

"Media Guide on Death and Dying," a descriptive listing of more than 200 film, tape, and slide programs available from American sources, can be obtained from:

Biomedical Communications
750 Third Avenue
New York, N.Y. 10017
U.S.A.

Film Strips / Tapes or Records

A Time for Everything / Death, #4 in the series "Discovering God's Creative Goodness." F.S. / Tape 6 minutes. Suitable for all ages (separate adult and children's scripts).

Available from:

Holt, Rinehart and Winston Ltd.
55 Horner Avenue
Toronto, Ontario M8Z 4X6

Loss and Grief S121 A series from which the following are related to Dying. F.S. / Tapes or Records.

#1 *Loss* 25 minutes
#2 *The Grief Process* 29 minutes
#3 *When Someone is Grieving* 33 minutes
#4 *The Child who Left Us* (Leukemia) and
Portrait of Peter (Down's Syndrome) 11 minutes

Instruction manual available. Available from:

Concept Media
P.O. Box 19542
Irvine, C.A. 92714
U.S.A.

Perspective on Dying S107 Tapes or Records only.

#1 *American Attitudes Towards Death and Dying*
#2 *Psychological Reactions of the Dying Person*
#3 *Hazards and Challenges in Providing Care*
#4 *Guidelines for Interacting with the Dying Person*
#5 *Viewpoint: The Dying Patient*
#6 *Viewpoint: The Nurse*

This series available with Instructor's Manual, packs of personal questionnaires and the book *Confrontations of Death.*
Available from same source as "Loss and Grief."

Coping with Death and Dying A series of five tapes only by Elisabeth Kübler-Ross.

Available from:

Ross Medical Associates
1825 Sylvan Court
Flossmoor, Ill. 60422
U.S.A.

If I Should Die Before I Wake, a Christian look at death, dying and grief. A course of 6 (weekly) studies with tape, guidebook and response sheet booklet, including also overhead transparencies.

Available from:

David C. Cooke Publishing Co.
850 North Grove Avenue
Elgin, Ill. 60120
U.S.A.

Films

All are 16 mm. The figure after the title gives the length in minutes.

Available from the National Film Board of Canada

Coming and Going 58 C.B.C. Film.
A visit to the palliative care unit at St. Boniface Hospital, Winnipeg, where terminally ill people are provided with a caring environment and prepared to meet death with dignity.

The Last Days of Living 58.
A film about the palliative care unit at the Royal Victoria Hospital, Montreal.

Death of a Gandy Dancer 26.
A 10 year old boy, and his family, learn to cope with the illness and death of his grandfather. Also availble from the Canadian Film Institute and from Marlin Motion Pictures Ltd. (see below for address).

Available from the Canadian Film Institute
B 20–75 Albert Street
Ottawa, Ontario K1P 5E7

Death and Mourning 60.
The staff of a residential treatment centre help the children express their grief over the sudden death of a staff member and all the other losses they have suffered.

A Documentary of Death 20.

Gift of Life / Right to Die 15.
An examination of medical ethics involved in a range of problems from euthanasia to transplant operations. The definition of death by "flat" EEG (cessation of brain waves) is explained.

Available from Visual Education Centre
75 Horner Avenue (Unit 1)
Toronto, Ontario M8Z 4X5

Come, Take my Hand 25.
The support that terminal cancer patients need in order to face death.

What Man Shall Live and Not See Death? 57
Dr. Kübler-Ross interviews a dying mother and helps the patient talk about preparing her youngest child for the coming loss.

Where is Dead? 19.
A 6 year old girl's reactions to the death of her 10 year old brother.

Available from International Telefilm Enterprizes
47 Densley Avenue
Toronto, Ontario M6M 5A8

Detour 13.
A woman of 83, dying in a large hospital. Modern medicine struggles to keep her alive as she struggles to die in peace.

The Magic Moth 22.
Raises, through the questions of a young boy about the death of his sister, many of the issues which concern us all.

Available from Holt, Rinehart and Winston
55 Horner Avenue
Toronto, Ontario M8Z 4X6

Science-New Frontiers: Extending Life 15.
Increasing life expectancy has raised questions about the nature of man and the meaning of life. When do we have the right to extend life and when to let death take its course? Who will determine who should be saved?

Available from the B.B.C., Manulife Centre
55 Bloor Street (Suite 510)
Toronto, Ontario M4W 1A5

Marek 47.
This child dies after an open heart operation. The film is about the courage of his family at this time of crisis.

Available from Canadian Filmmakers Distribution Centre
144 Front Street West (Suite 430)
Toronto, Ontario M5J 1G2

Moments in Between 58.
As members of a hospital team for two years, the filmmakers were able to record the thoughts and feelings of five terminally ill patients.

Available from Ralph Ellis and Associates
556 Church Street
Toronto, Ontario

Whose Life is it Anyway? 53.
A quadriplegic patient asks the hospital staff to let him die with dignity. They refuse on the grounds that he is not able to make a rational decision. He hires a lawyer and a court hearing decides the issue.

Available from Bruce Raymond Ltd.
63 Huntley Street
Toronto, Ontario M4Y 2L2

To Die with Dignity 25.
A Miami doctor's proposal to withdraw life support machines and drugs from incurable patients.

Available from Novalis-Select
P.O. Box 998
Oakville, Ontario L6J 5E8

To be Aware of Death 15.
The film creates an environment which makes it easy to discuss the subject of death.

Available from Marlin Motion Pictures Ltd.
47 Lakeshore Road East
Mississauga, Ontario L5G 1C9

The Death of Ivan Ilych 28.
From the series "Begin with Goodbye." Leader's guide and bibliography available. A dramatization of Tolstoy's classic short story. At the end a number of people with life threatening illness respond to what they have seen and discuss their own feelings.

A Dose of Reality 16.
From the T.V. Program "60 Minutes." This deals with the anticipation of dying and what one nurse is doing to help terminally ill patients.

How Could I Not be Among you? 28
A portrait of a young poet who has been told he has six months to live and how he learned to live each day for the things he loved and valued.

The Right to Die 56.
The questions which face the terminally ill, mercy killing, suicide and the medical prolongation of life are examined through discussions with patients. The Living Will is introduced.

Grief Therapy 19.
From the T.V. Program "60 Minutes." A clinical psychologist treats a mother who is suicidal and grief stricken 2-1/2 years after the death of her 12 year old daughter. After therapy sessions for a week, she comes to accept this death.

A Time to Cry 28.
From the series "Begin with Goodbye." Leader's guide and bibliography available. Two episodes. In one, a mother of three young children and her husband cope with her impending death from cancer and the children are told everything. In the other, a minister's wife learns to cope after his death.

Very Good Friends 29.
From the series "Learning to be Human." How a 13 year old girl copes with the sudden death of her younger sister.

Available from the American Journal of Nursing Film Library
c / o Association-Sterling Films
600 Grand Avenue
Ridgefield, N.J. 07657
U.S.A.

Until I Die 30.
Dr. Kübler-Ross examines the stages through which patients generally progress when they learn of approaching death. An interview with a cancer patient illustrates her methods and a conference with staff who observed the interview indicates their reactions to the patient's comments.

Available from University of California Extension Media Centre
Berkeley, C.A. 94720
U.S.A.

Who Should Survive? 26.
The case history of a Down's syndrome baby with intestinal obstruction which could have been corrected surgically but who died after 15 days because the parents refused consent. Filmed at Johns Hopkins Hospital, Baltimore. A panel discusses the ethical, legal and scientific issues involved.

Available from Horizons in the Life Cycle Inc.
(Filmmakers Library Inc.)
290 West End Avenue
New York, N.Y. 10023
U.S.A.

Death — Dying in a Hospital 43.
A portrait of a man dying from cancer at Calvary Hospital, New York. It initiates discussion of feelings about death and how to assist the dying patient.

Dying 90.
Composed of three documentaries which portray three differing ways of dealing with death.

Last Rites 30.
The mystery of death and its incomprehensibility to a child.

Planting Things I Won't See Flower 26.
A family struggling with the demands forced on them by the impending death of the mother.

Resource Materials

Reading Packets, Institute of Society, Ethics and the Life Sciences, 360 Broadway, Hastings-on-Hudson, New York 10706, U.S.A.

Packet 200: Care of the Dying — Cultural and Personal Dimensions
Packet 300: Death and Dying — Definition of Death
Packet 400: Death and Dying — Euthanasia, Allowing to Die and Refusal of Treatment
Packet 500: Death and Dying Survey Packet

National Hospice Organisation, 301 Tower Suite 606, 301 Maple Avenue West, Vienna, Va. 22160 U.S.A.

Euthanasia Educational Council, 250 West 57th Street, New York, N.Y. 10019 U.S.A.

Study Guide

Introduction

This report has been produced as a document for study and discussion. In this section five outlines are given for people in parishes who wish

— to become more familiar with ideas presented in the report
— to identify and share personal concerns and anxieties about death and dying
— to clarify moral issues associated with death and dying

Here are designs for five sessions. These can be adapted and used more than once. Discussion will uncover many new questions that can be picked up at future sessions.

1 Action — Reflection — Action
2 A Moral Dilemma
3 A Statement of Principle
4 A Hard Case — a role play
5 Questions Posed by the Report

1 Action — Reflection — Action

Everyone knows something about death. We have all had experience of it, even though the experience is different for each person and for each group of people. Because the authors think it important not to theorize about death, at least at the beginning of a study, the first design begins with a serious consideration of the experience of participants in a group.

There are five steps. First, people are asked to tell their own story and then are invited to think critically about its meaning for them: to move from "what" to "why." After describing and reflecting on their own experience, the story of the Christian community is brought to bear, through the selection of scripture or other parts of the Christian tradition. Participants are then asked, "What does The Story say to your story?" "In the light of your own experience, how do you make The Story yours and begin to live out its message?" (The term *dialectic* is used instead of *dialogue* to indicate that this is not just a conversation back and forth but a critical reaction.) Finally, group members identify their future action in light of the vision of God's kingdom and their own practice. How will they act in the future?

The timing in the accompanying design is approximate but is also generous in order that people may take seriously the task of sharing. These are the phases of a procedure for "acting-reflecting" on death and dying. In a group of 8 to 10 people the following steps can be taken in the whole group. For larger gatherings people can work in groups of 3 or 4 and report their findings. While strong feelings may surface, it is worth remembering that this is a learning group, not a therapy group. Probing is inappropriate. Encourage people to share.

a *Share your Story* - Describe an experience of a death (relative, friend, loved one, enemy) that was significant for you. (very difficult, positive, etc.) Take 5 minutes by yourself to write silently. Share. *(30 mins.)*

b *Critical Reflection* - What consequences has this event had for you? What would you like to be different? Why? Reflect on this silently, jot down thoughts, then share. *(20 mins.)*

c *Christian Story* - Ask someone to prepare a *short* reflection on verses from the Burial Office of the Prayer Book page 591, 1 Corinthians 15, Romans 8:14–39, John 6:35–40, John 10:10, or some other passage which holds up the vision of resurrection. It is helpful if this presentation is made from a personal perspective in dialogue — "and that's my telling of it" rather than "and that's the way it is." *(10 mins.)*

d *Dialectic* - What does this story and your experience say to you? How does the gospel relate to your experience? What questions does it raise? Is the gospel story helpful, unhelpful? What do you think about resurrection? What do you think of the quotation from H.A. Williams (p. 60). *(30 mins.)*

e *Vision* - How do you think things will be in the future? Do you think you will act, think, feel differently? Is there some action we need to take as a group, or as individuals? Are there questions or issues that need to be explored further? *(30 mins.)*

2 A Moral Dilemma

Many of our moral questions arise because of the conflict we experience between different moral values. The report examines some of these conflicts from the theological, medical, legal, and economic points of view. When values are in conflict and we experience dilemma, our basic "moral stance" is used to "arbitrate" or "referee." In other words, we are required to exercise judgment. Only seldom can the simple application of rules or laws provide an unambiguous solution. In the end we must judge what is the right or wrong thing to do and try to give reasons for — justify — what makes an action right. This is not easy! Few of us can give clear concise statements about deeply held convictions or ultimate commitments.

One method for articulating these commitments was developed by Dr Lawrence Kohlberg of Harvard University in his research on moral development. A brief story is presented which describes a dilemma. People are asked to make a judgment — "Do this or do that?" — and give a reason — "Why?" The emphasis is always on the question, "What would make it right to do so and so?" Gradually we are pushed to identify for ourselves the commitments that influence our moral judgments. One of Kohlberg's moral dilemmas is used here in an adapted form.

Note — If the group is small enough (under 8 people), each question could be discussed as it is posed by a leader. If the group is larger, it would be helpful for a leader to ask people to write out and discuss their answers in groups of 3 or 4 before reporting to the larger group after question 7 and again after question 9. Finally ask the group — in 3 or 4s — to summarize by listing the principles they used to make judgments about life and death issues.

A man is near death from a special and rare form of cancer. No drugs work, there is no other treatment that can save his life, and the doctor expects that he has but a few months to live. He is in terrible pain and is so weak that a good dose of pain killer may make him die sooner. He is often delirious, but in calm periods he begs the doctor to give him enough to kill him. He says that he can't stand the pain and is going to die anyway.

1 Should the doctor do what he asks and give him the drug that may hasten his death? Why?

2 Does the man have the right to decide what to do with his own life in this case? Why?

3 Would you blame the doctor in any way for giving him the drug? Why?

4 Suppose he asked his wife to administer a lethal injection. Is she in the same moral position as the doctor? Why?

5 Would a "good" spouse commit such an act? If she weren't particularly close or affectionate, would this make any difference?

6 Would it be right for a doctor to hasten the death of a suffering person if such practice were not against the law? What would make it right, wrong?

7 Should the law permit or prohibit euthanasia?

The doctor finally decides to hasten the man's death to put him out of his pain. He does it against the law. The police find out and he is brought up on a charge of murder. The jury finds him guilty even though they know the man asked for death.

8 What sentence should the judge give? Why?

9 Should the doctor have been acquitted? Why?

3 A Statement of Principle

If a group has worked on the issues at least once before, this design could be used for formulating a moral point of view on one of the more critical issues in the paper.

Ask participants to work silently by themselves on completing this sentence.

I believe that it is right / wrong to hasten the death of a child born with gross and uncorrectable neurological defects. It is right / wrong to practise active euthanasia / passive euthanasia because . . . *(5–10 mins.)*

Ask people to move around the room and try to find three or four others whose reasons are most like theirs. Suggest: Don't be hasty, and don't agree too early; probe for differences. This is not a contest. *(20 mins.)*

Ask each group to develop a statement of their point of view and report it to the other groups. Write it on newsprint if that's possible. *(30 mins.)*

From their own perspective, each group should reflect on the statements of the other groups. Ask them to focus on — "The points I find helpful in the statements of others." "The points I find unhelpful in the statements of others." Discuss. *(30 mins.)*

4 A Hard Case

Through a role play — which may be defined as "a spontaneous portrayal (acting out) of a situation by selected members of a learning group" — people usually come closer to experiencing the feelings and attitudes connected with a problem than they do by reading or hearing an account of it. This role play is designed to enable people to consider some of the moral questions related to a decision about death and dying. The roles can be varied somewhat by the leader of the group — for example, parents positively want the surgery and the doctor doesn't. The leader's job is to pick the role players, brief the audience about its role, keep time, "de-role" the actors, and lead the discussions afterwards.

Role Play — In some cases of Down's Syndrome it is common for the patient to have a bowel obstruction that will lead to death if untreated. Some doctors recommend against this simple surgery in these cases. Ask four people to play the parts of doctor, parents, and chaplain. This is their first conversation of any substance. All that the parents know is that "something is wrong!"

The Doctor — knows that prospects for successful surgery are excellent but that the patient will be retarded to an unknown degree. He is inclined to perform the surgery.

The Parents — are of course shocked and distraught. They try to consider all the possibilities and are deeply aware of their own limited emotional and financial resources. They are inclined not to consent to the surgery. They would like more time but there isn't any.

The Chaplain — will try to support the parents in whatever decision they make. He believes the child's life should be preserved, but he knows he personally will not have the continuous care of the child through the years.

The Task — to decide whether or not to have the surgery done.

Note — the characters do not need elaborate roles, but it is important not to choose people for whom the role would be "loaded" (too close to life).

Give the characters names and write them on a large badge which the characters wear. Ask other participants to choose a character to observe and to summarize the principles on which the character based his / her decision. Let the role play run long enough for several issues to be considered. A good rule of thumb is "two crises" — that is, let it run past two occasions when you would be tempted to stop it. It will usually pick up! When you top it, de-role as follows.

1 Ask each character in turn to describe his / her experience, both feelings and thoughts — "What is it like to be the doctor, etc?"

2 Remove the name tags and ask them to join the groups.

3 Group discussion — observers should report their observations. When referring to the characters, the third person and the character's name should be used, rather than the "real" name ("The father was upset when" not "You were upset when").

De-roling sometimes takes longer than you think. As group leader, be attentive to a character stuck in a role. More talking about the role is usually an answer to being "stuck."

If these questions are not thoroughly discussed, introduce them in the group discussion: Are the parents *obliged* to consent to the surgery? If the parents do not consent and the doctor were to apply to the courts for an order to do the surgery, who should be obliged to care for the child? What role can the church play?

5 Questions Posed by the Paper

A number of questions are raised in the report itself. These are listed here along with some others as possible discussion questions for a group. No doubt others will have been raised by participants.

1 Ask participants to identify those points in the report at which they began to feel uneasy, angry, argumentive, excited, or disappointed. What questions come out of these?

2 Ask people to write down the first word that comes to mind when the following phrases are used — image of God, sanctity of life, quality of life. What does ''sanctity of life'' mean to people? ''What must a person do or be in order for us to recognize the presence of God in that person?'' (p. 19).

3 ''To avoid slow physical deterioration and the prolonged misery of the family, would some form of active euthanasia be compatible with compassion for the patient and family and with respect for the past life and dignity of the patient?'' (p. 40).

4 As you think about it, what would be a ''fair and easy passage'' for your own dying? What three things do you fear the most about your own death?

5 Are there steps regarding the health–care system (sickness-care?) in your community that you would like to take?

6 Who should decide about stopping life support systems? Some think the doctor, others the courts, others a tribunal in the hospital. What do you think?

7 ''It has been said that the moral worth of a society can be judged by the protection and care it gives to its weak and helpless members . . . Are we willing to accept higher taxes to eliminate consideration of cost in the ordinary care of seriously sick and dying patients?'' (p. 57). To what extent should economics be a consideration in the care of the dying? Should this group take some further action in the local community?